Fine Structure of Human Cells and Tissues

TATSUO EBE, M. D.
Departments of Anatomy and Internal Medicine
Niigata University School of Medicine, Niigata, Japan

SHIGERU KOBAYASHI, M. D.
Associate Professor, Department of Anatomy
Niigata University School of Medicine, Niigata, Japan

A Wiley-Interscience Publication

JOHN WILEY & SONS INC. New York · Toronto
IGAKU SHOIN LTD. Tokyo

Library of Congress Catalog Card Number: 72-4340

ISBN: 0-471-22941-5

Printed and bound in Japan

FOREWORD

Since the day of ANDREAS VESALIUS, the knowledge of the normal structure of the human body has been the basis of medicine. In the field of ultrastructure research, which has developed in the past two decades, our knowledge of cells and tissues is still much based on or even restricted to findings on mice, rats and other experimental animals. The fine structure of the human body, as the light microscopic and macroscopic structures do, conspicuously deviates in certain points from that of animal bodies, while in certain other points it strikingly corresponds to the latter. Both discrepancy and accordance deserve to be demonstrated exactly.

Knowledge of the fine structure of the *normal* human body is now especially indispensable, as technical advances in biopsy have made possible the examination of the ultrastructure of almost every organ and tissue of the patient's body and the detection of pathological changes under the electron microscope has become, in some cases, critically important for the diagnosis and treatment of the patient.

Now that only one relatively small atlas of the human ultrastructure (R. P. LAGUENS and C. L. A. GÓMEZ DUMM: Atlas of Human Electron Microscopy, 1969) is available, as far as I know, the publication of this atlas treating almost all important tissues and cells systematically and comprehensively is timely and is expected to be useful for students and researchers.

Dr. EBE, senior author of this book, is a physician at the University Hospital of Niigata. Besides his clinical duties, he has been engaged for eight years in electron microscope studies, especially of the kidney and lung, in the Department of Anatomy. Dr. KOBAYASHI, the other author, has been one of the leading members of the electron microscope research group in the Anatomy Department and his main interest of study has been the digestive tract and endocrine system. Other members of this research group have helped the authors by contributing micrographs of various tissues.

I am very glad to point out that this atlas is thus the result of the endeavor and enthusiasm of two young authors and the friendship of their colleagues. This book, born in a small medical school on the northern coast of Japan, will be widely used by medical students and researchers all over the world.

September 1971

TSUNEO FUJITA, M. D.
Professor and Director
Department of Anatomy
Niigata University School of Medicine
Niigata, Japan

PREFACE

During the past two decades, the development of the electron microscopic techniques has brought about such important and abundant information on the fine structure of organisms that more or less major changes have become inevitable in the teaching of histology and cytology in medical and dental schools. It has become common for students, during the course of their education, to study in some way electron micrographs of various cells and tissues.

Although many excellent electron microscopic atlases have been published, most of them deal mainly with such laboratory animals as the rat, the mouse and the guinea pig. We believe that medical and dental students should be, as far as possible, educated by using human materials, because their future object is man himself. This atlas was intended to cover the essential items concerning the fine structures of the human body. All micrographs appearing in this atlas are of human material. We hope this atlas will be useful not only for students but also for the researchers who are just beginning the study of the fine structure of human cells and tissues.

It was in 1964 that we initiated the electron microscope studies under the guidance of Prof. TORAO YAMAMOTO, the former Director of the Anatomy Department at the Niigata University School of Medicine. At that time, the hard frontier age in electron microscopy, had ended, and the methods for specimen preparation, such as glutaraldehyde and osmium tetroxide fix-ation, epoxy resin embedding, microtomy and electron-staining with heavy metals had been established. We were able to master these modern techniques within a relatively short time. In the course of this training, our interest was not focused on specific cells and tissues, but we intended to obtain general knowledge on the fine structure of the human body. In this period we prepared more than fifteen thousand electron micrographs; about one-third of these are of human material. In 1969, Prof. TSUNEO FUJITA, successor of Prof. YAMAMOTO as the Director of our Anatomy Department, suggested that we publish a selected series of electron micrographs of human materials in the form of a concise atlas. Without encouragement and support from him, we doubt whether this book would have been started or completed. More-over, he read the entire text in manuscript form and pointed out errors in the content. We express our cordial thanks to Prof. FUJITA.

Since our collection of electron micrographs was insufficient for a book, we made good the deficiency by borrowing excellent electron micrographs from our colleagues in the Niigata University. Particularly, we are grateful to Dr. HIDEHIRO OZAWA, Associate Professor of Anatomy in the Dental School, who willingly co-operated, supplying many original electron micrographs of the tooth, bone, epidermis and so forth. Our thanks are also due to Dr. MASAYUKI MIYOSHI, Associate Professor of Anatomy in the Medical School, for the helpful criticism and encouragement throughout the writing of this work and for supplying electron micrographs of ejaculated spermatozoa. Furthermore, we acknowledge the following colleagues in the Medical School: Dr. AKIRA HATTORI, Department of Internal Medicine, for electron micrographs of blood and bone marrow; Drs. KENICHI KANO and YASUO TOGAWA, Depart-ment of Urology, for electron micrographs of the male reproductive system and adrenal cortex; Dr. HIROSHI MATSUKURA, Department of Forensic Medicine, for electron micrographs of the thymus. We also acknowledge Prof. KAZUMASA KUROSUMI and Dr. NORIOMI BABA, Institute of Endocrinology in the Gunma University, for supplying an electron micrograph of a lactating mammary gland. Finally, we owe very much to Mrs. VIRGINIA DEFFNER, an American librarian who lives in Niigata city, because our English was ultimately checked by her.

September 1971

TATSUO EBE
SHIGERU KOBAYASHI

CONTENTS

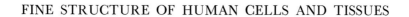

FINE STRUCTURE OF HUMAN CELLS AND TISSUES

CONNECTIVE TISSUE

Mast cell

Mast cells are widely distributed in connective tissue and often tend to congregate along small blood vessels. Their cytoplasm is filled with intensely metachromatic granules which are known to contain heparin, histamine (and serotonin in the rat and the mouse) and some proteolytic enzymes. Thus, they influence the blood-clotting mechanism, vasoconstriction and capillary permeability, and play an important role in the local inflammatory process.

Top: A mast cell and a blood capillary.

This electron micrograph shows a mast cell and a blood capillary in the lamina propria of the gastric mucosa.

The nucleus of the mast cell is round and the chromatin appears to be more compact at the periphery than in the center. The cell surface is covered by numerous microvillous projections (p). The Golgi complex (Go) is well developed and the granular endoplasmic reticulum (Er) is inconspicuous. Mitochondria (m) are small and scarce.

The cytoplasmic granules (g) of the mast cell range in diameter from 0.25 to 1.5 μ and are limited by a membrane sac. They are often irregular in outline and usually heterogeneous in appearance. They generally contain different components forming lamellar whorls, crystalline materials and so forth. Thus, the cytoplasmic granules are often referred to as "compound granules."

The blood capillary consists of a fenestrated endothelial cell with a small nucleus, a continuous basal lamina and an adventitial cell.

c:	Centriole.
Cf:	Collagenous fibril.
Clu:	Capillary lumen.
Ed:	Capillary endothelial cell.
Nu:	Nucleolus.
Par:	Parietal cell.

Gastric fundic mucosa of a 21-year-old male patient. Biopsy material obtained for diagnostic purpose by means of a fiber gastroscope. Phosphate-buffered 2.5% glutaraldehyde fixation followed by 1.3% osmium tetroxide post-fixation. Uranyl acetate and lead tartarate staining. ×18,000.

Bottom: High power electron micrograph of mast cell granules.

Lm: Limiting membrane.

Surgically-obtained subcutaneous tissue of the abdominal skin from a 39-year-old female with cholelithiasis. Fixation is the same as the top picture. Uranyl acetate and lead citrate staining. ×140,000. (Photograph courtesy of Dr. H. Ozawa)

REFERENCES:

Fedorko, M.E. and J.G. Hirsch: Crystalloid structure in granules of guinea pig basophils and human mast cells. J. Cell Biol., *26*: 973–976, 1965.

Weinstock, A. and J.T. Albright: The fine structure of mast cells in normal human gingiva. J. Ultrastr. Res., *17*: 245–256, 1967.

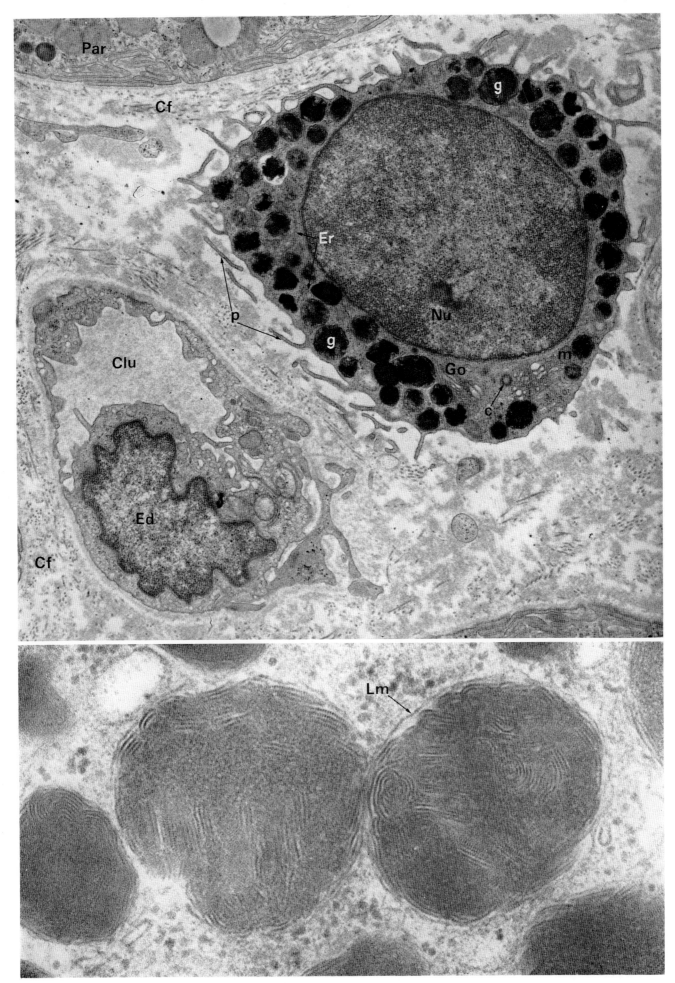

3

CONNECTIVE TISSUE

Plasma cell

It is widely accepted that the plasma cell is the producer of antibodies. This cell occurs frequently in the lamina propria of mucous membrane, though it is extremely rare in the common connective tissue.

The cell is round or oval in shape. The nucleus has an eccentric position, is round and contains one or more well-developed nucleoli (Nu). Chromatin masses characteristically are gathered to the nuclear envelope forming the cartwheel figure of the nucleus of this cell. The cytoplasm is to a large extent occupied by sacs of granular endoplasmic reticulum (Er), usually arranged in parallel and concentric patterns. The sacs of granular endoplasmic reticulum are usually narrow, though they may be distended as shown in this picture. In the middle of the cell are seen centrioles (c), around which are Golgi complexes (Go), mitochondria (m) and lysosomes (Ly). This area is called cell center or centrosome.

The presence of extensive granular endoplasmic reticulum is a characteristic feature of protein-producing cells. By the use of the immunohistochemical technique, recent investigations of the plasma cell have revealed that antibodies are present in the cisterns of granular endoplasmic reticulum.

From the lamina propria of the pyloric antrum of a 53-year-old male. Biopsy material obtained under direct vision by means of a fiber gastroscope. Immersion fixation with phosphate-buffered 2.5% glutaraldehyde followed by post-fixation with 1.3% osmium tetroxide solution. Doubly stained with uranyl acetate and lead tartarate. ×27,000.

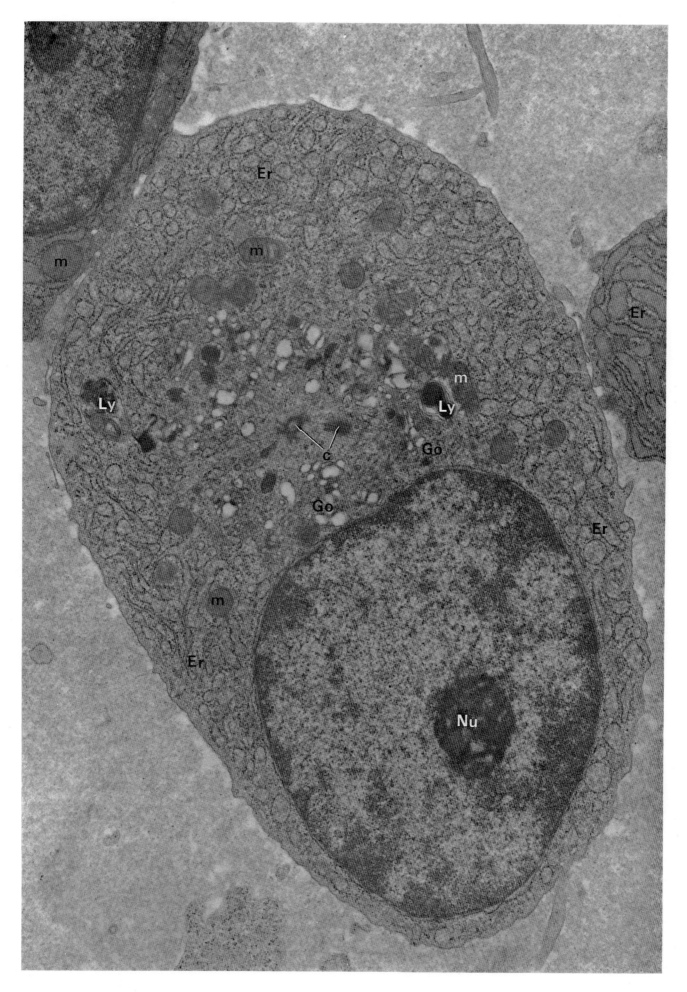

5

Cell center of the plasma cell (Top)

In most cells the cell center is an area close to the nucleus and contains two centrioles (diprosome). Many microtubules radiate from this area, around which mitochondria and Golgi complexes are generally gathered. This area as a whole is believed to play an important role as a kinetic center during cell division.

The plasma cell is known to have a prominent cell center. Two centrioles (c) are seen in the center of this electron micrograph. Small masses of dense materials or centriolar satellites (arrows) are closely associated with them. They are surrounded by prominent Golgi complexes (Go) consisting of numbers of small vesicles and parallel-arranged, smooth-surfaced cisterns filled with a fine granular substance. Mitochondria (m) and granular endoplasmic reticulum (Er) are situated around the clusters of Golgi complexes. Small, membrane-bound, round granules (Ly) seen among Golgi complexes are considered to be of lysosomal nature. Numerous microtubules (t) are seen radiating from the cell center to the periphery of the cell.

Cross section of a centriole seen in the plasma cell (Top right)

A centriole is a hollow cylindrical structure of $0.2\,\mu$ in diameter, 0.3–$1.0\,\mu$ in length, consisting of nine triplets of microtubules of about 250Å in diameter. The triplets are parallel to each other and, in cross section, are located at the apex of a regular nonagon.

The basal bodies of flagella and cilia are morphologically identical to centrioles.

Russell body of the plasma cell (Bottom)

Plasma cells occasionally accumulate granular masses in well-developed cisterns of their granular endoplasmic reticulum. They correspond to the Russell bodies of light microscopy, which signify the beginning of the degeneration of the cell.

In this picture, four Russel bodies are shown. They are represented by round and homogeneous bodies (g) of medium electron density within the lumen of the granular endoplasmic reticulum. They have no limiting membrane, but are always distant from the membrane of granular endoplasmic reticulum (Er).

N: nucleus.

All three pictures cited on this page are from the same material as that of the picture on page 5. Top: ×41,000. Top right: ×160,000. Bottom: ×30,000.

REFERENCE:

SHIGEMATSU, T.: The fine structure of various types of myeloma cells as revealed by electron microscopy. Arch. histol. jap., *30*: 375–400, 1969.

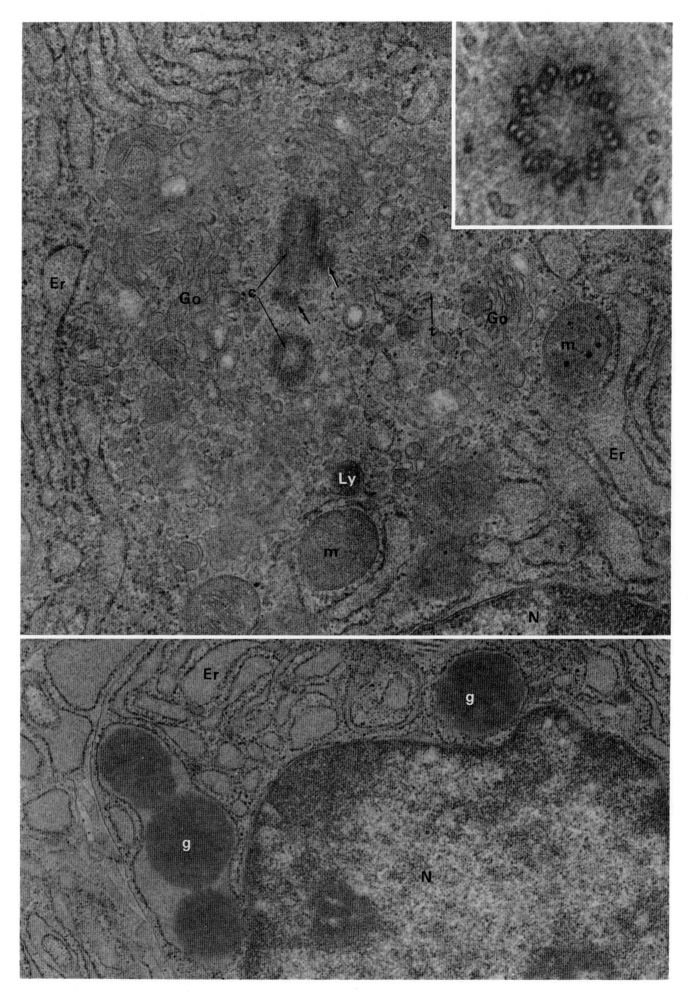

7

CONNECTIVE TISSUE

Histiocyte

The histiocyte is an element of the reticuloendothelial system, sometimes called the macrophage system. It can take up, by pinocytosis, particulate matters such as bacteria, dead cells and foreign bodies. It has the ability to migrate and to play an important role in the site of an inflammation.

The histiocyte is irregular in outline, but there are no microvillous projections on the cell surface. Like other connective tissue cells, it forms neither desmosome nor tight junction with neighboring cells. The nucleus is usually irregular in shape and often contains round inclusion bodies (Ib). The ample cytoplasm is characterized by an abundance of lysosomes of high electron density (Ly). They are variable in size and shape and are limited by a single membrane. They are known to contain various kinds of hydrolytic enzymes which serve in the digestion of phagocytized matters. Golgi complexes (Go) near the nucleus are composed of stacks of cisterns and numbers of small vesicles. Mitochondria (m) are mainly located around the Golgi complexes. Strands of smooth-surfaced endoplasmic reticulum (Ser) are scattered among the lysosomes. Cisterns of granular endoplasmic reticulum often show parallel array and are situated in the periphery of the cell.

c : Centriole.
Cf : Collagenous fiber.
N : Nucleus.
Pc : Plasma cell.
∗ : Matrix of the connective tissue.

Material and method are the same as those of the picture on page 5. ×17,000.

REFERENCE:

ATHANASSIADES, T. J., L. HERMAN and G. R. HENNIGAR: Electron microscopy of cytoplasmic inclusions within "macrophages" of human tissue. Lab. Invest., *14*: 409–423, 1965.

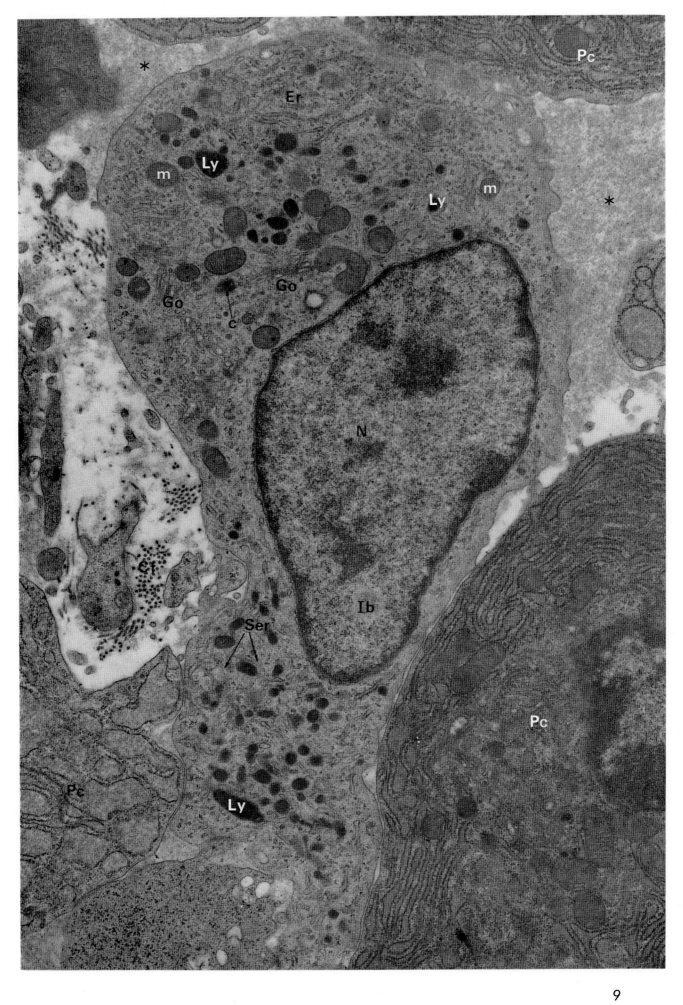

9

CONNECTIVE TISSUE

Fibroblast and fibrocyte

The fibroblasts are the most common cells in all forms of fibrous connective tissue. As their name implies, they elaborate connective tissue fibers and also form some of the amorphous ground substance. The fibrocytes are essentially mature fibroblasts which have ceased their active protein synthesis. They become active following tissue injuries.

Top : This survey picture of a portion of the mucous membrane of the oviduct shows a basal portion of the epithelium and a part of the connective tissue lining it. The epithelium is separated from the connective tissue by an undulating basal lamina (Bl). Fibrocytes (Fc) in the connective tissue have long cytoplasmic processes which run parallel to the epithelial base. Between fibrocytes are seen numerous collagenous fibers (Cf) cut at different angles. They consist of bundles of thin collagenous fibrils. The matrix of the connective tissue contains amorphous material of low electron opacity (∗). A profile of a blood capillary containing an erythrocyte (R) and a portion of a venule (Ven) are seen respectively in the lower left and in the lower right corner.

Eo : Epithelium of the oviduct.

Bottom : A closer view of the upper micrograph showing the fibrocytes and collagenous fibers in a fibrous connective tissue. The fibrocytes are characterized by the dense nucleus (N), long and thin cytoplasmic processes and scarcity of cell organelles.

The site with the large arrow corresponds to that in the top picture.

Ld : Lipid droplet.

Top and Bottom : The oviduct of a 33-year-old female. Obtained by operation (salpingectomy for prevention of conception). Phosphate-buffered 2.5% glutaraldehyde fixation followed by 1.0% osmium tetroxide post-fixation. Uranyl acetate and lead tartarate staining. Top : ×5,000. Bottom : ×11,000.

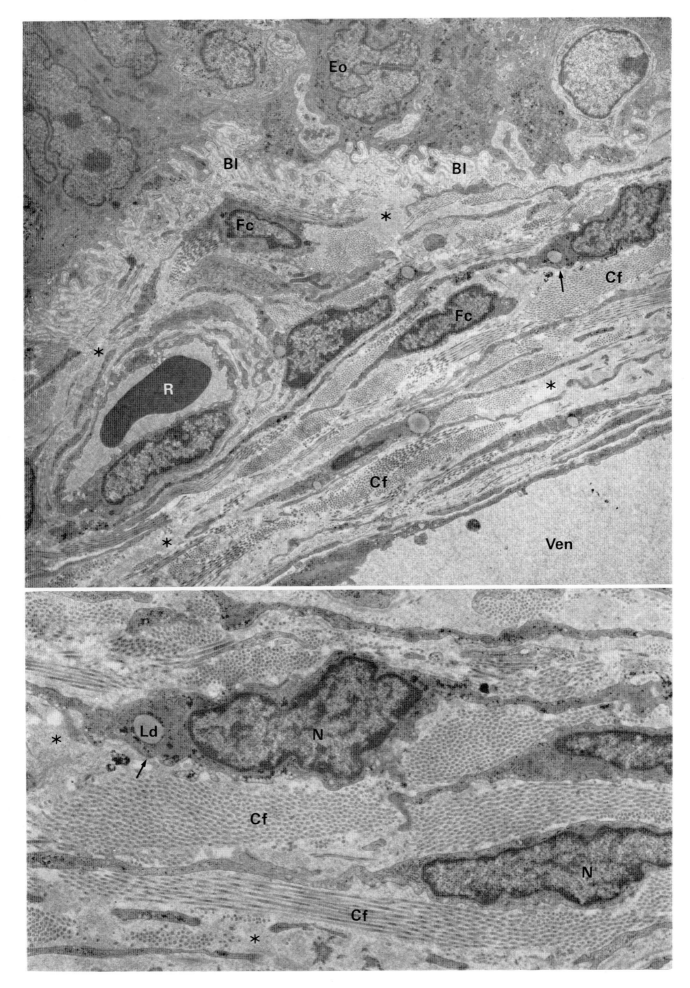

Fibroblast (Top)

Unlike the fibrocyte, the fibroblast contains abundant cisterns of granular endoplasmic reticulum and well-developed Golgi complexes in its cytoplasm. The intercellular space is filled with bundles of collagenous fibrils (Cf) and microfibrils which are believed to be precursors of thick collagenous fibrils.

Bmf : Bundle of microfibrils.
Cf : Bundle of collagenous fibrils.
Er : Granular endoplasmic reticulum.
Go : Golgi complex.
m : Mitochondrion.
N : Nucleus.
v : Caveola intracellularis.
* : Coated vesicle suggesting the pinocytotic activity of the cell.

From the interstitial tissue of the lung of a 57-year-old male patient with pulmonary fibrosis. Open lung biopsy for diagnostic purpose. Cacodylate-buffered 2.5% glutaraldehyde fixation followed by post-fixation with 2.0% osmium tetroxide in the same buffer. Lead tartarate staining. ×45,000.

Fibrous lamina in the nucleus of fibrocyte (Bottom)

The fibrous lamina is a thin layer of filamentous material on the inner aspect of the nuclear envelope (arrows) and is known to be especially conspicuous in the fibrocyte.

Cy : Cytoplasm.
Im : Inner nuclear membrane.
Kp : Karyoplasm.
Np : Nuclear pore.
Om : Outer nuclear membrane.
r : Ribosome.

From a mesenterial lymph node of a 61-year-old male with esophageal cancer. Obtained by operation. Phosphate-buffered 2.0% glutaraldehyde fixation followed by post-fixation with 2.0% osmium tetroxide solution. Uranyl acetate and lead tartarate staining. ×100,000.

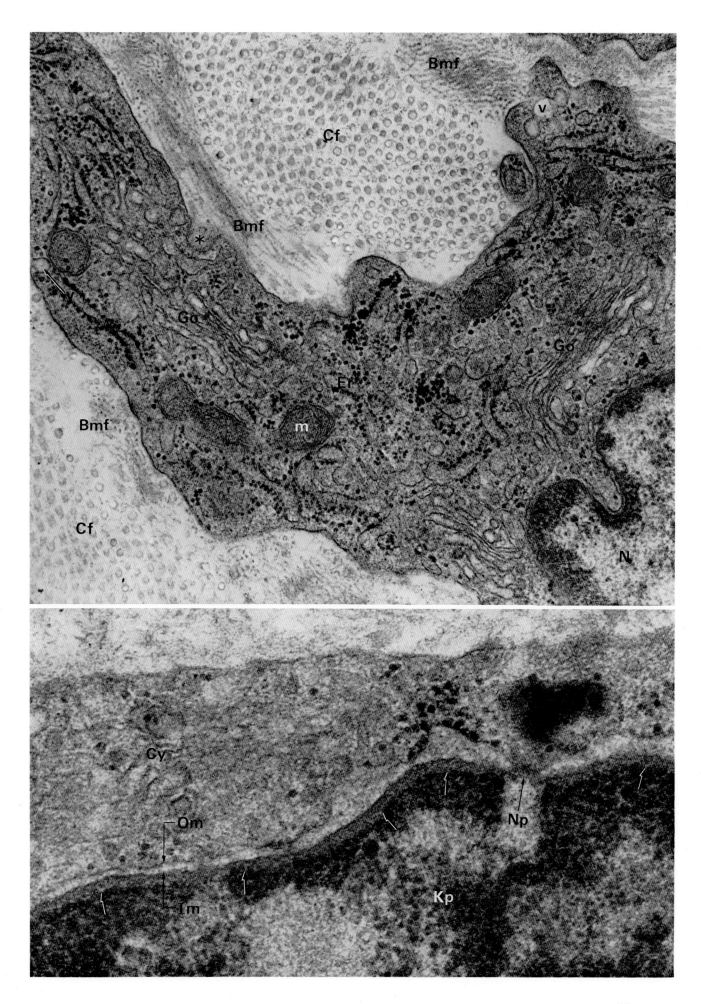

13

CONNECTIVE TISSUE

Collagenous fiber

Collagenous fibers are widely distributed in all types of connective tissue. They possess little elasticity, but offer great resistance to a pulling force. They are easily dissolved by weak acids, and yield gelatin when boiled.

Collagenous fibers consist of bundles of collagenous fibrils which are held together by inter-fibrillar substance. Collagenous fibrils are characterized by periodic crossbanding at intervals of 640Å. Within each 640Å banding, there are several additional bands called intraperiodic bands.

Chemical analysis showed that the collagenous fibrils are composed of a protein containing large amounts of hydroxyproline, glycine, proline and so forth. These amino acids are linked together to form a molecular chain. Three such chains are united by hydrogen bonds to constitute a tropocollagen molecule which measures about 2,800Å in length and about 14Å in diameter. A collagenous fibril is formed of many tropocollagen molecules aligned side by side in a staggered fashion.

Top : Cross section of a collagenous fiber. The unit fibrils of collagen measure about 600Å in diameter here, but it is known that, among different tissues, they vary greatly in diameter. A much finer fibrous element seen in groups near the collagen fibrils is assumed to represent the reticular fiber seen in the light microscopy. A basal portion of an epithelial cell with a basal lamina enters the right upper corner of this micrograph.

Bl : Basal lamina.
Cf : Collagenous fiber.
Rf : Reticular fiber.

From the lamina propria of the gall bladder of a 39-year-old female with cholelithiasis. Obtained by cholecystectomy. Method is the same as that of the pictures on page 11. ×75,000.

Bottom : Collagenous fibrils in a longitudinal section. Note the characteristic major period (arrows) measuring about 640Å, and a repeating pattern of crossbanding within it.

From the ovary of a 48-year-old female. Obtained by operation. Method is the same as that of the pictures on page 11. ×105,000.

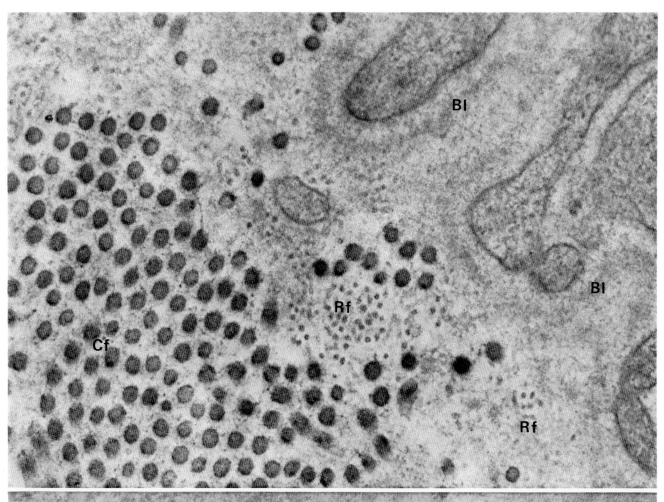

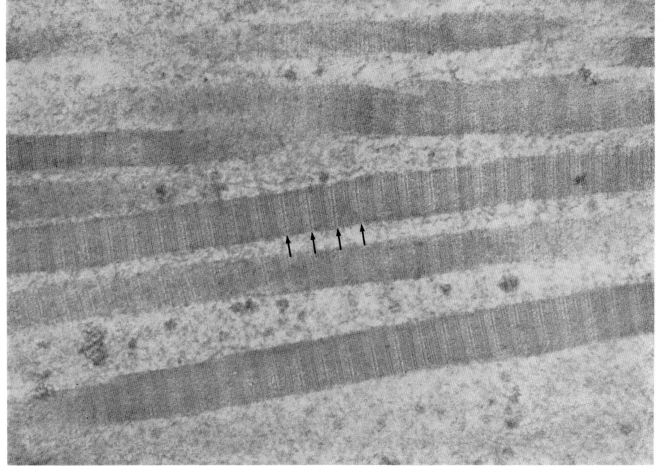

15

Elastic fiber

Elastic fibers are much less frequent in most types of connective tissue than are collagenous fibers. They occur in the form of fibers or granules as well as in sheets. Their main component is elastin, a yellow albuminoid containing large amounts of glycine, proline and valine. They show a greater resistance to boiling, as well as to dilute acids and alkalis, than do the collagenous fibers. As their name implies, their most important characteristic is their elasticity.

The main part of an elastic fiber looks like a homogeneous mass of a medium electron density. The surface of each mass is covered by thin filaments with a diameter 50 to 60Å. These filaments seem to form a continuous network about the fiber to bind them into bundles. Within the homogeneous mass of the elastic fiber, fusiform or fibrillary dense areas are scattered (arrows). At high magnification these areas are seen to contain thin fibrils similar to those covering the surface of the mass.

Top: Longitudinal section of elastic fibers.

From the auricle of the heart of a 16-year-old male with tetralogy of Fallot. Obtained by operation. Cacodylate-buffered 2.5% glutaraldehyde fixation followed by 1.3% osmium tetroxide post-fixation. Uranyl acetate and lead tartarate staining. ×17,000.

Bottom: Cross section of elastic fibers and a portion of a mast cell.

- Ef: Elastic fiber.
- Fc: Cytoplasmic process of fibrocyte.
- g: Mast cell granule showing concentrically arranged fingerprint-like pattern of substance.
- N: Nucleus.
- p: Microvillous projection of the mast cell.

From the lamina propria of the bronchus of a 72-year-old male patient with lung cancer. Obtained by operation. Phosphate-buffered 2.5% glutaraldehyde fixation followed by 2.0% osmium tetroxide post-fixation. Uranyl acetate and lead citrate staining. ×90,000. (Photograph courtesy of Dr. H. Ozawa)

REFERENCE:

CHARLES, A.: Human elastic fibres. Electron microscopic appearance of the elastic fibres of human skin in thin sections. Brit. J. Dermatol., *73*: 57–60, 1961.

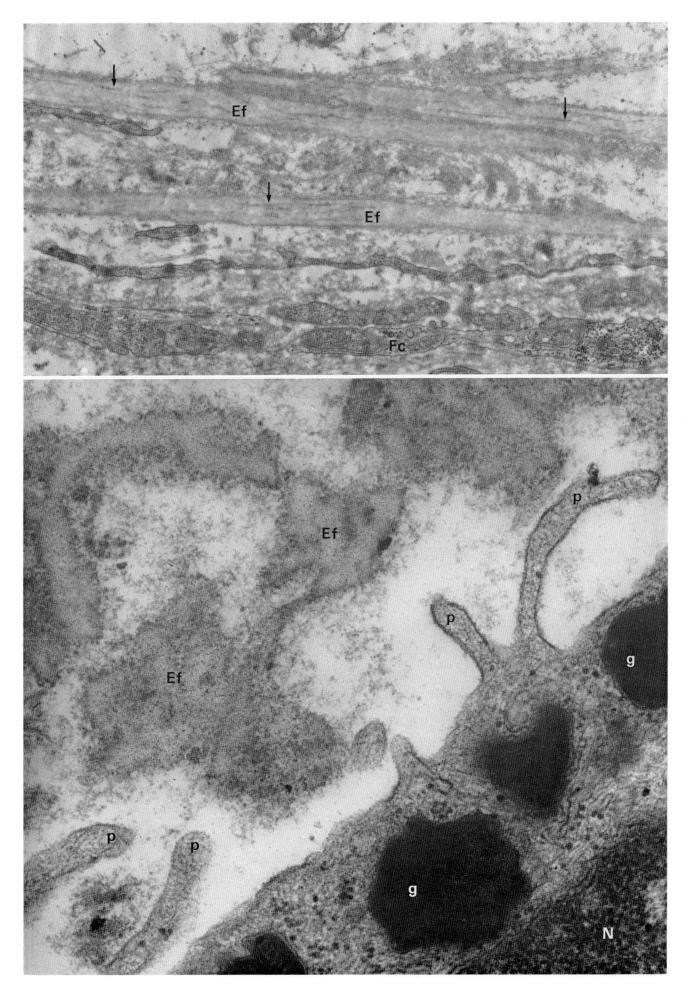

17

Fat cell

The mature fat cell is so large, ranging up to $100\,\mu$ in diameter, that it is hard to take the whole of its profile in an electron micrograph. Immature fat cells, which are smaller in size, are shown in this atlas. By the huge lipid droplet growing in the cytoplasm during the differentiation of the cell, the nucleus is (N) pressed to one side, while the cytoplasm is reduced to a thin rim retaining small Golgi complexes, small mitochondria (m) which are either spherical or filamentous in shape, scattered profiles of granular endoplasmic reticulum, free ribosomes and abundant cytoplasmic filaments. The lipid droplet is not enclosed by a membrane.

Cf : Collagenous fiber.
Fb : Fibroblast.
Ld : Lipid droplet.
Nu : Nucleolus.

Top and Bottom: Young fat cells from the subcutaneous tissue of a 6-month fetus (♀, 600g). Phosphate-buffered 2.5% glutaraldehyde fixation followed by post-fixation with 1.0% osmium tetroxide solution. Lead tartarate staining. Top: ×5,000. Bottom: ×9,000.

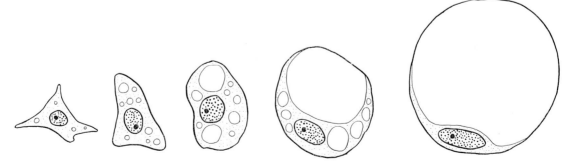

Diagrams showing the development of fat cells: The fat cells originate from undifferentiated cells resembling fibroblasts. In an early stage of the cell's development, many lipid droplets occur in the cytoplasm. Then the lipid inclusions increase in size and coalesce to form a single droplet of large size.

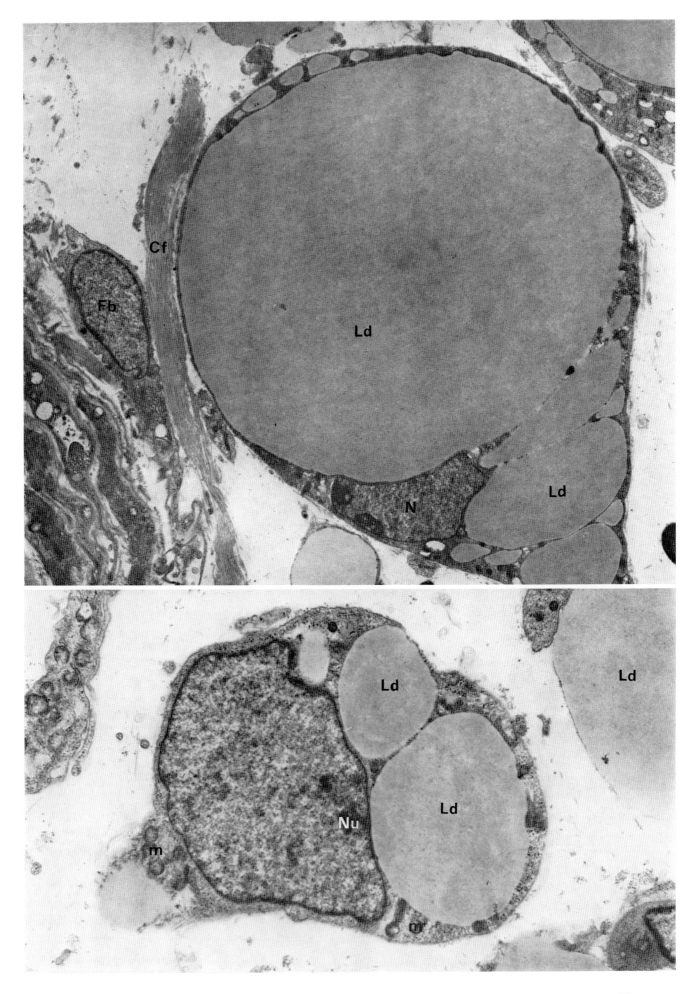

CARTILAGE TISSUE

Cartilage is a special type of dense connective tissue. Like other connective tissues, it consists of three elements: cells, fibers and ground substance. Together, the latter two elements constitute the matrix or intercellular substance which provides both the rigidity and the resilience of cartilage.

Cartilage is classified into three subtypes depending upon the fibers predominating in the matrix: hyaline cartilage predominated by collagenous fibers, elastic cartilage specialized by added elastic fibers, and fibrous cartilage which is considered to be a transitional form between cartilage and dense connective tissue. The ground substance of cartilage is mainly a complex of chondromucoid, a mucoprotein rich in chondroitin sulfate. The cartilage cells or chondrocytes are thought to elaborate fibers as well as the ground substance of cartilage.

Fetal hyaline cartilage (Top and Bottom)

In early fetal life, most of the skeleton is temporarily formed of hyaline cartilage. Electron micrographs shown on page 21 were obtained from a developing finger bone of a 6-month human fetus. The cartilage cell has a large nucleus of oval profile (N). The cytoplasm contains a well-developed Golgi complex (Go), cisterns of granular endoplasmic reticulum (Er), mitochondria (m), glycogen (Gl) and large vacuoles (Va). In the cartilage matrix, tangles of collagenous fibrils are seen. Small dense particles scattered between collagenous fibrils are thought to be of chondromucoid nature.

Ma: Matrix.
Nu: Nucleolus.

Top and Bottom: Fetal hyaline cartilage from a developing finger of a 6-month fetus (♀, 600g). Phosphate-buffered 2.5% glutaraldehyde fixation followed by post-fixation with 1.3% osmium tetroxide solution. Uranyl acetate and lead tartarate staining. Top: ×12,000. Bottom: ×39,000.

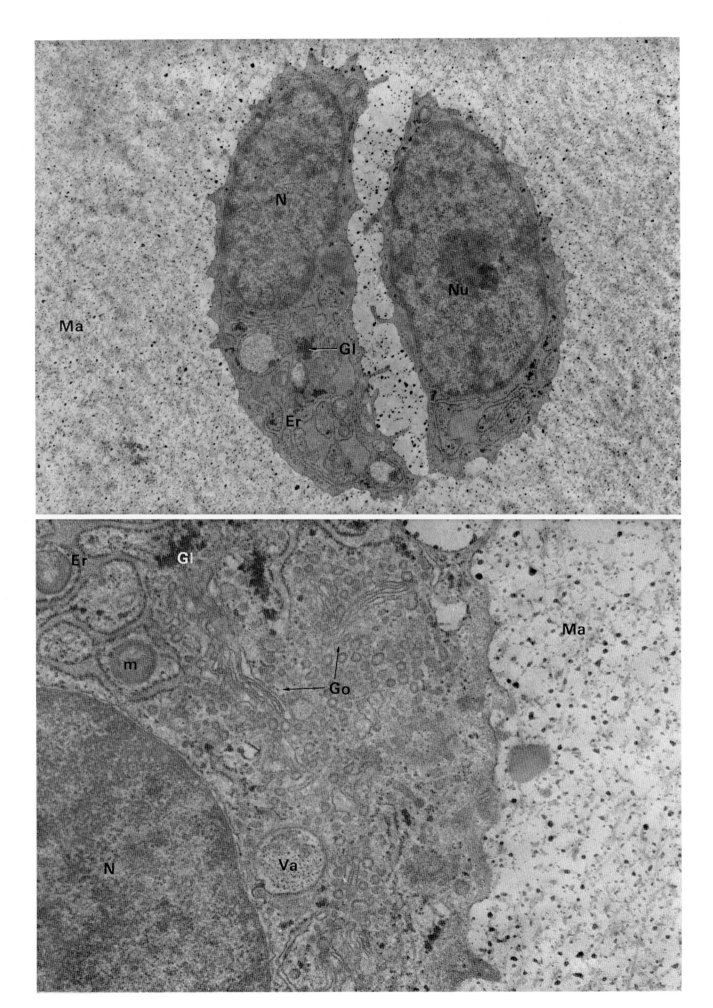

BONE TISSUE

Bone cells and bone matrix

Bone constitutes most of the skeleton, except in early fetal life. Bone consists of matrix and cells. The bone matrix contains fibers, chiefly collagenous, and a ground substance containing large amounts of inorganic salts including calcium phosphate, calcium carbonate, calcium fluoride and magnesium fluoride. Fibers in the bone matrix contribute to the strength and resilience of bone, whereas inorganic salts are responsible for the hardness and rigidity. The bone cells are classified into three types: osteoclast, osteoblast and osteocyte. These cells are closely interrelated in function and readily transform from one type to the other.

Top : Osteoclast.

The osteoclast is a large multinuclear cell engaged in the absorption and removal of the bone substance. Its rich cytoplasm contains a number of mitochondria (m), strands of granular endoplasmic reticulum (Er), lysosomes (Ly) and multi-locular Golgi complexes (Go). The surface of the cell, especially where it is in contact with the bone, is provided with numerous cytoplasmic processes (p) which are believed to play an important role in bone absorption.

    Cf :   Collagenous fiber.
    N :   Nucleus.

Developing finger bone of a 7-month fetus (♀, 800g). Fixation with 2.5% glutaraldehyde followed by 1.0% osmium tetroxide post-fixation in phosphate buffer. Uranyl acetate and lead tartarate staining. ×6,500.

Bottom : Osteoblast

The osteoblast produces the organic bone matrix and some enzymes needed for the process of calcification.

In this picture profiles of two osteoblasts are shown. They have morphological features which are characteristic of cells actively engaged in protein synthesis; i.e., a well-developed granular endoplasmic reticulum (Er) and prominent Golgi complexes (Go). The bone appears black owing to the density of the mineral salts in its matrix. Note the upper right corner where non-mineralized bone matrix (Nbm) is seen.

    Cbm :   Calcified bone matrix.
    N :   Nucleus.
    ∗ :   Cell boundary.

Developing mandible of a 7-month fetus (♂, 1,850g). Phosphate-buffered 2.5% glutaraldehyde fixation followed by 1.0% osmium tetroxide post-fixation. Uranyl acetate and lead citrate staining. ×10,000. (Photograph courtesy of Dr. H. Ozawa)

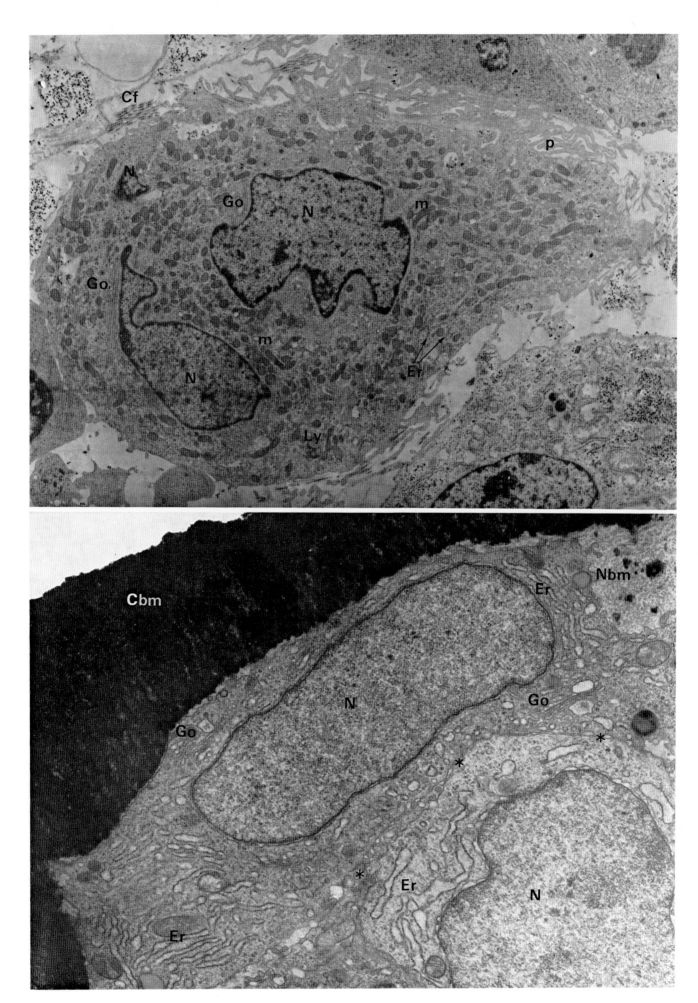

23

BONE TISSUE

Osteoblast and forming bone matrix

The cytoplasm of the osteoblast is occupied mainly by cisterns of granular endoplasmic reticulum (Er) which are usually distended with the products of synthesis. Adjacent to the nucleus there is a cell center in which a centriole (c) and well-developed Golgi complexes (Go) are seen. The Golgi complex is associated with numerous vacuoles (Va) containing fine granular material. Arrows indicate coated vesicles, suggesting pinocytotic activity of the cell. From the area immediately beneath the surface, cell organelles such as mitochondria and granular endoplasmic reticulum are excluded.

In the upper right corner of this micrograph is the calcified bone matrix (Cbm), subjacent to which is a number of collagenous fibrils of newly-formed, unmineralized bone matrix.

       m : Mitochondrion.
       N : Nucleus.
       * : Cell boundary.

Developing mandible of a 7-month fetus (♂, 1,450g). Phosphate-buffered glutaraldehyde fixation followed by osmium tetroxide post-fixation. Uranyl acetate and lead citrate staining. ×45,000. (Photograph courtesy of Dr. II. Ozawa)

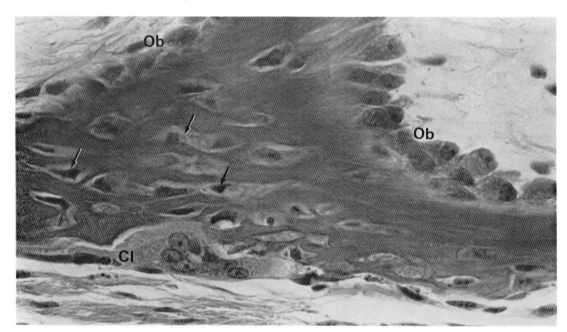

Photomicrograph of a newly formed spicule of the bone: Osteoblasts with darkly stained cytoplasm are arranged along the surface of the newly-formed bone (Ob). Some of them have become imprisoned in the bone matrix and have differentiated into the osteocytes (arrows). An osteoclast (Cl) with several nuclei occupies the shallow pit of the spicule which is located at the surface opposite to that covered by a layer of osteoblasts.

From developing parietal bone of a 15-week fetus (♀, 130g). Bouin fixation. Hematoxylin and eosin staining. ×750.

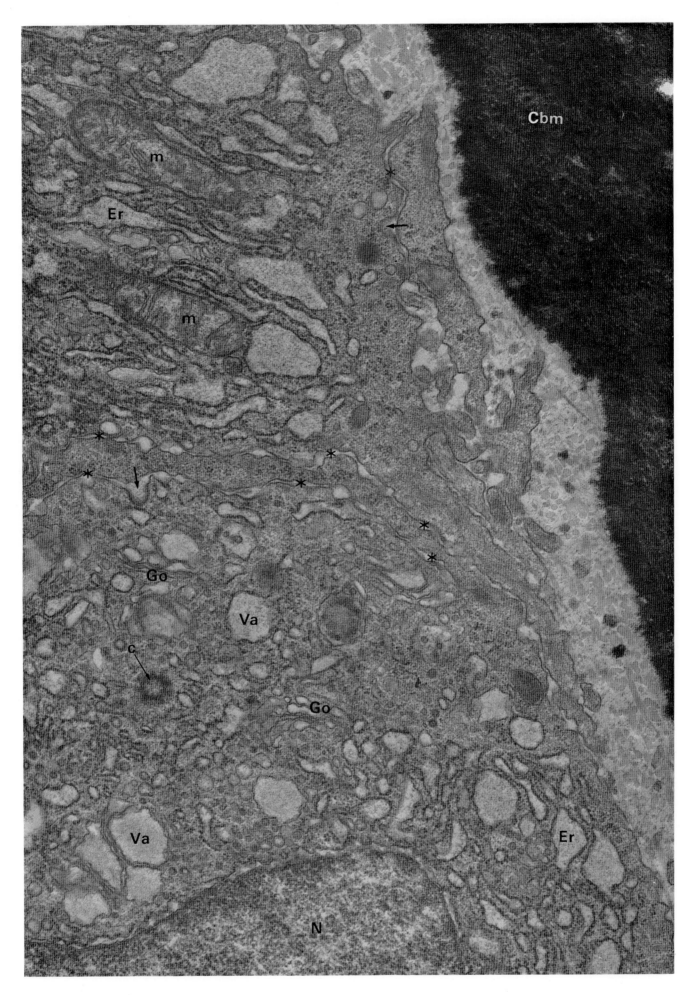

25

BONE TISSUE

Osteocyte in its lacuna (Top)

An osteocyte, the principal cell of the bone, is an osteoblast which has been enclosed in the developing matrix of the bone. Thus, osteocytes and osteoblasts have much the same morphological features, though the granular endoplasmic reticulum is less developed in the osteocyte.

In the osteocyte shown in this photograph, the outline of the cell is irregular and several cytoplasmic processes are seen. The nucleus (N) is large in size and deeply indented (arrow). The relatively rich cytoplasm contains cisterns of granular endoplasmic reticulum (Er), large mitochondria (m), cytoplasmic microtubules and several dense bodies (Ly).

Cbm : Calcified bone matrix.
Cf : Collagenous fibril.
Cv : Coated vesicle.
N : Nucleus.
Um : Uncalcified matrix of bone.

Material and method are the same as those of the picture on page 25. ×16,700. (Photograph courtesy of Dr. H. Ozawa)

Mineralized bone matrix (Bottom)

Apatite crystals of various shapes are seen.

Developing rib bone of a 7-month fetus (♂, 1,850g). Method is the same as that of the picture on page 25. ×120,000. (Photograph courtesy of Dr. H. Ozawa)

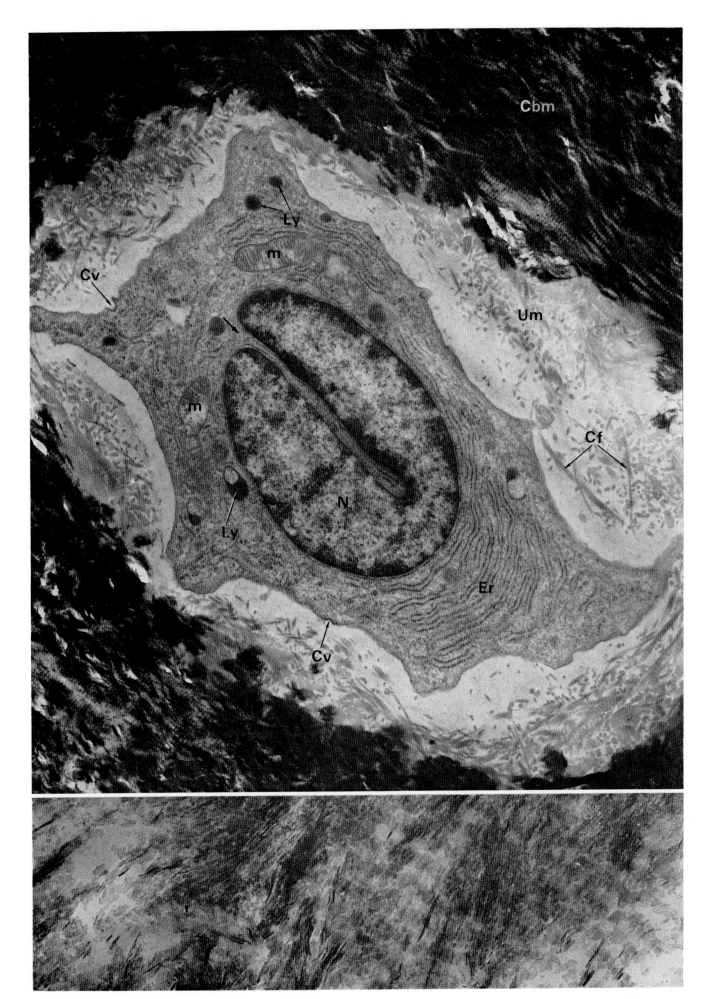

27

BLOOD VESSEL

Arteriole

The arteriole is a small-calibered artery situated immediately before the capillaries. Its wall consists of endothelial cells resting on a thin elastic membrane (tunica intima), a single layer of smooth muscle cells (tunica media) and a connective tissue sheath (tunica adventitia). The smooth muscle of the arterioles plays an essential role in the regulation of blood flow in the capillary.

This micrograph shows a cross section of an arteriole seen in the muscularis of the stomach. The lumen of this arteriole (Alu) is lined by two endothelial cells, which are closely attached to one another by a junction (j). The cell swells into the lumen at the portion of the nucleus (N). Numerous vesicles (v) occur in the cytoplasm near both lumal and basal surfaces. From the base of the endothelial cell, slender cytoplasmic processes (Cp) extend into the sub-endothelial space to surround, outside of the innermost leaf of the basal lamina (Bl), the proper endothelial cell.

A sickle-shaped smooth muscle cell is shown with a pair of centrioles (c) near the nucleus (N). The cytoplasm contains ample myofilaments and some mitochondria (m). A few lamellar layers of the basal lamina (Bl) are interposed between the endothelium and the smooth muscle layer.

A connective tissue layer composed of the basal lamina beneath the smooth muscle and collagenous fibers (Cf) embedded in the amorphous substance surrounds the former two layers. In this presumable terminal portion of the arteriole the internal elastic membrane seems not developed.

Fc : Fibrocyte.
Gl : Glycogen particle.
Mm : Smooth muscle cell of the muscularis.
R : Erythrocyte.

Biopsy material obtained from the pyloric antrum of a 51-year-old male. Phosphate-buffered 2.0% glutaraldehyde fixation followed by post-fixation with 1.0% osmium tetroxide solution. Uranyl acetate and lead tartarate staining. ×20,000.

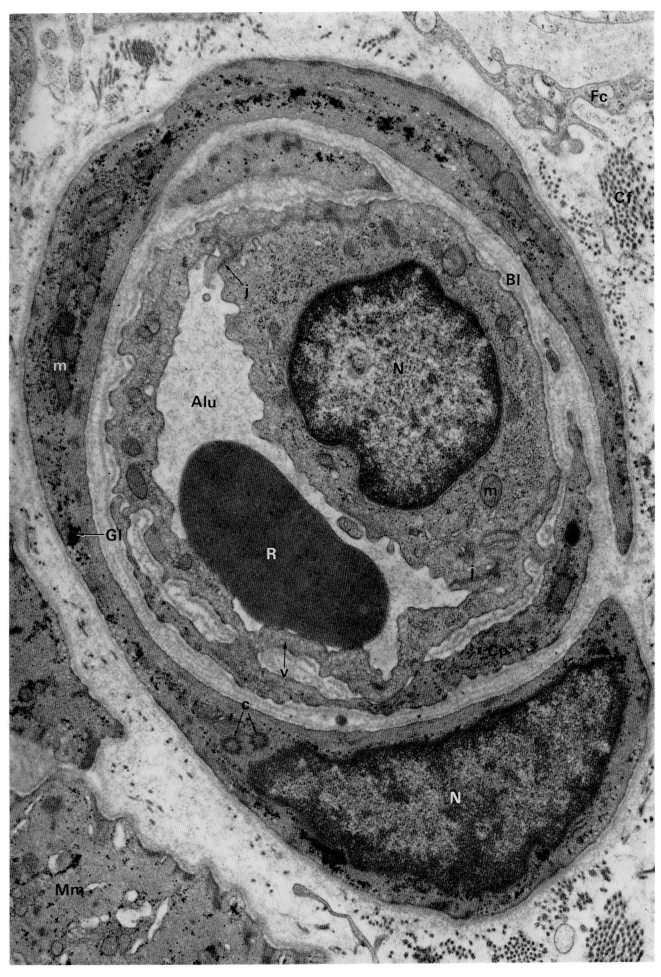

29

Blood capillary

Blood capillaries are the site where substances are exchanged between blood and tissue fluid. Their wall generally consists of three layers: endothelium, basal lamina and adventitia. The capillary endothelium is a simple squamous epithelium with little, if any, intercellular cleft and it forms the main filter which is semi-permeable and selects substances passing through. The basal lamina (Bl) is apparently similar to that of other epithelia. It supports the endothelial tube from its outside and is believed to serve as a barrier against relatively coarse particulate matters. The adventitial layer consists of pericytes (Pc) and connective tissue fibers and is not important as a barrier to the passage of substances as compared with the previous two layers.

Capillaries seen in the gastro-enteric mucosa, kidney, endocrine glands and some other tissues are characterized by an extremely attenuated endothelium having numerous fenestrations, or pores, of 700 to 800Å in diameter (arrows). This type of blood capillary is called "visceral type" as distinguished from the capillaries seen in muscular tissues, the cerebral cortex and in various other tissues. In these tissues, the capillary endothelium is relatively thick and has no fenestrations. These capillaries are called "muscular type."

Cf: Collagenous fiber.
Clu: Capillary lumen.
Fc: Fibrocyte and its process.
j: Junction between two endothelial cells.
Mf: Muscle fiber.
N: Nucleus of an endothelial cell.

Top: Capillary of visceral type seen in the lamina propria of the gall bladder.

Surgically-obtained gall bladder of a 39-year-old female with cholelithiasis. Phosphate-buffered 2.5% glutaraldehyde fixation followed by 1.0% osmium tetroxide post-fixation. Uranyl acetate and lead tartarate staining. ×11,000.

Bottom: Capillary of muscular type seen in the M. gastrocnemius.

Biopsy material obtained for diagnostic purpose from a 50-year-old female with idiopatic edema. Fixation with s-collidine-buffered 2.5% osmium tetroxide. Lead tartarate staining. ×8,000. (Photograph courtesy of Dr. A. HATTORI)

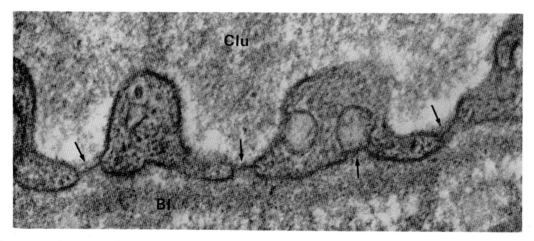

High-power electron micrograph of a fenestrated capillary wall: Fenestrations of an endothelial cell and small invaginations of its plasma membrane (caveolae) are closed by a diaphragm with a central knob (arrows).

From surgically-obtained duodenal mucosa of a 69-year-old male with gastric cancer. Phosphate-buffered 2.5% glutaraldehyde fixation followed by 1.0% osmium tetroxide post-fixation. Uranyl acetate and lead citrate staining. ×135,000. (Photograph courtesy of Dr. H. OZAWA)

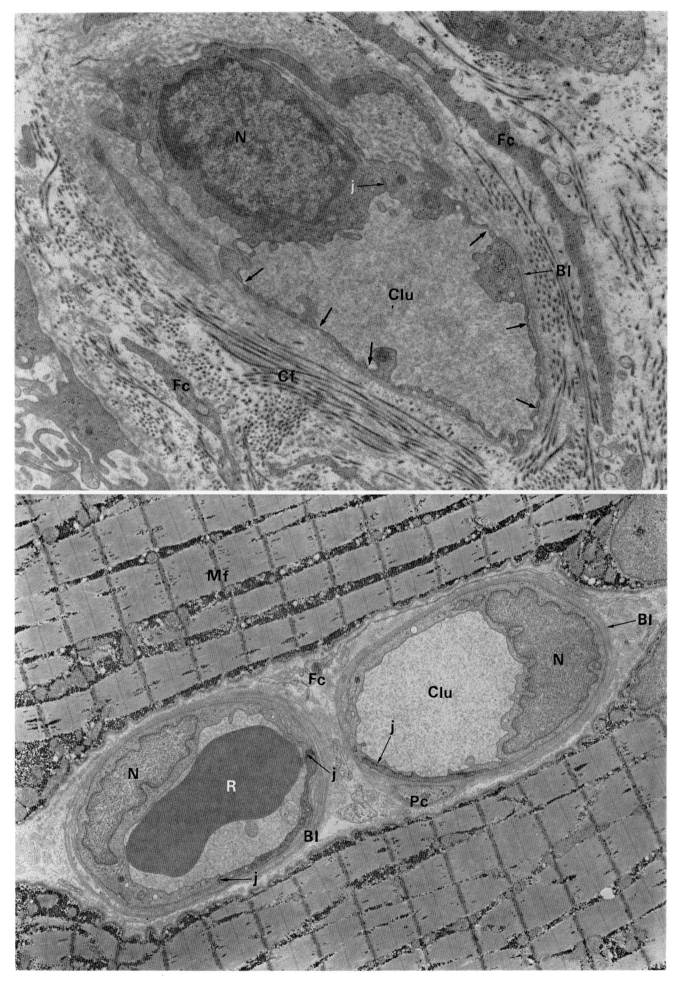

31

BLOOD VESSEL

Venule

The venule is the smallest vein and is the transitional vessel from the capillary to the venous system. It has a wide lumen surrounded by a thin wall composed of a squamous endothelium, basal lamina and a small amount of connective tissue.

Top: Venule in the submucosa of the stomach. The endothelial cells (Ed) have a flat and irregularly-shaped nucleus (N) and contain a few cell organelles such as mitochondria, dense bodies and granular endoplasmic reticulum. A basal lamina (Bl) runs beneath the endothelial layer. Attenuated cytoplasmic processes (Cp), presumably from pericytes or smooth muscle cells, are beneath the basal lamina and are also sandwiched between its divided leaves. A part of these processes seems to be issued from the endothelial cell itself as shown in the upper left part of this micrograph (arrow).

Cf: Collagenous fiber.
Pc: Plasma cell.
R: Erythrocyte.
Sm: Smooth muscle.
Vlu: Lumen of the venule.

Material and method are the same as those of the picture on page 29. ×8,500.

Bottom: Venule in the lamina propria of the urinary bladder. The endothelium (Ed) is surrounded by several layers of tortuous basal lamina (Bl) and slender cytoplasmic processes (Cp) of the pericytes. Within the lumen of the venule (Vlu), a number of leukocytes are contained.

Cf: Collagenous fiber.
Fc: Fibrocyte.
Lc: Lymphocyte.
Nl: Neutrophilic leukocyte.
R: Red blood cell.

From the uninvolved area around a tumor of the urinary bladder of a 63-year-old male. Cacodylate-buffered 2.5% glutaraldehyde fixation followed by post-fixation with 2.0% osmium tetroxide solution. Stained with lead tartarate solution. ×3,000.

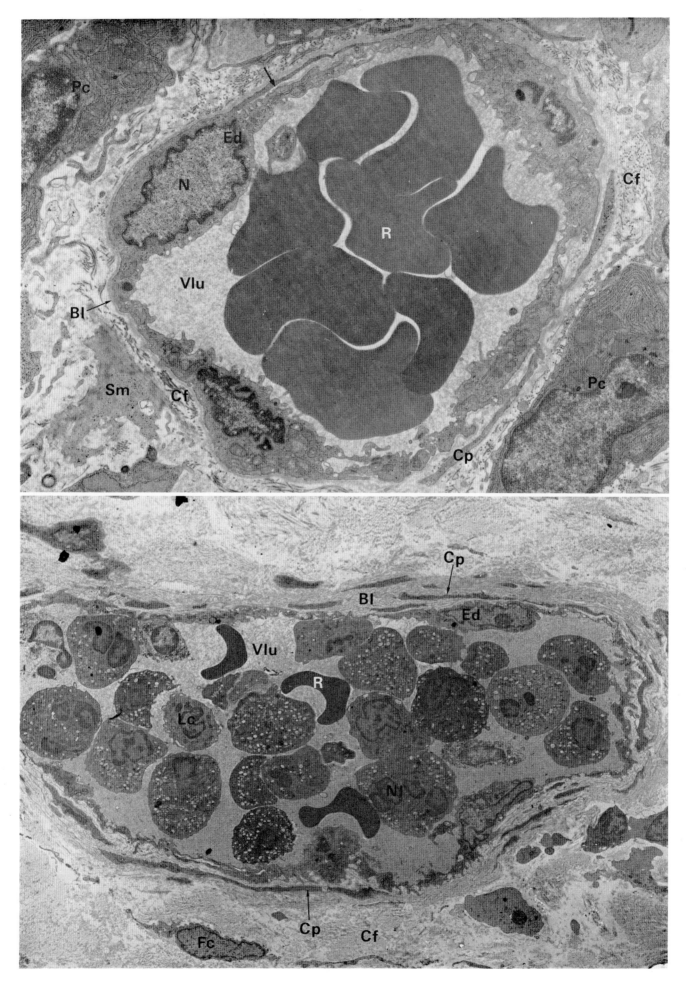

33

BLOOD VESSEL

Vein

The wall of the vein shown in this micrograph is composed of three layers. The tunica intima is a layer of endothelial cells (E) with a thin connective tissue or basal lamina (Bl) beneath it. These cells are poor in cell organelles and closely attached to each other by a junction (j). The tunica media is made of a single layer of circularly-arranged smooth muscle cells (Sm). Dense glycogen masses (Gl) occur in the cytoplasm. A basal lamina is also seen beneath this layer. The tunica adventitia is a thick layer of connective tissue consisting of longitudinally-arranged fibrocytes (Fc) and collagenous fibers (Cf). In the lower left corner, a vas vasorum (Vv) lined by a thin endothelium is seen.

Vlu: Lumen.

Vein in the tissue around the Zuckerkandl organ of a 7-month fetus (♂, 1,850g). Phosphate-buffered 2.5% glutaraldehyde fixation followed by 1.0% osmium tetroxide post-fixation. Uranyl acetate and lead tartarate staining. ×15,000.

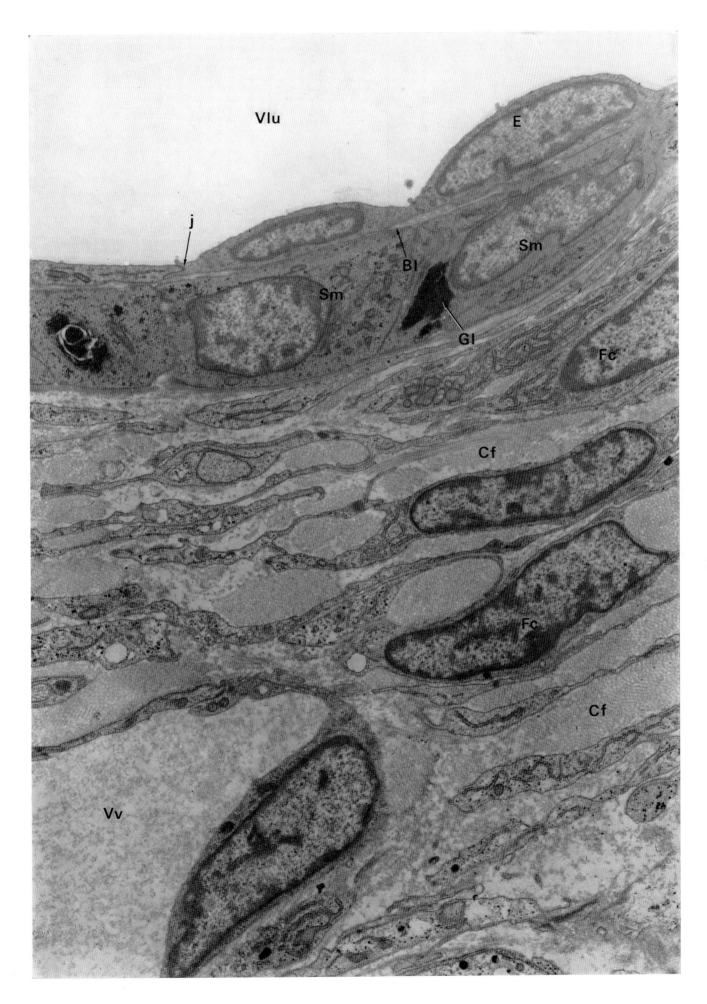

35

The leukocytes, or white blood cells, are divided into two categories, agranular and granular. Agranular leukocytes, comprising lymphocytes and monocytes, have cytoplasm which, in light microscopy, stains evenly with basic dyes, though faint azurophilic granules may often be found. The granular leukocytes or granulocytes are characterized by a content of numerous, obvious cytoplasmic granules. These cells are classified into three groups: acidophiles with granules which are stained with acid dyes, basophiles characterized by granules stained with basic dyes and neutrophiles containing fine granules which are tinged an intermediate color in a mixture of acidic and basic dyes.

Lymphocyte (Top)

Lymphocytes comprise 25 to 30 per cent of the leukocytes in the peripheral blood and vary in size from 8 to 15 μ in diameter.

The lymphocyte shown in this picture is roughly round in contour. Numerous, short cytoplasmic processes (p) are seen around the cell surface. The spherical or kidney-shaped nucleus has small nucleoli. Several mitochondria (m), a Golgi complex (Go), a centriole (c) and some microtubules (t) radiating from the cell center to the periphery are gathered on one side of the cell. Profiles of granular endoplasmic reticulum are not frequent, but free ribosomes are abundantly scattered throughout the cytoplasm. Two dense bodies (Db) which probably correspond to the azurophilic granules in light microscopy are contained in the lymphocyte.

Er : Granular endoplasmic reticulum.
Pl : Blood platelet.

From the peripheral blood of a 33-year-old male. Fixed in 1.0% glutaraldehyde followed by post-fixation with 2.0% osmium tetroxide solution in phosphate-buffer. Stained with uranyl acetate and lead tartarate solution. ×14,000. (Photograph courtesy of Dr. A. HATTORI)

Monocyte (Bottom)

Monocytes are the largest cells in mature leukocytes, measuring 12 to 18 μ in diameter and constituting 4 to 7 per cent of the leukocytes in the peripheral blood. They have an ability to phagocytize foreign matters and cell debris.

This micrograph shows a monocyte seen in the peripheral blood. The nucleus (N) appears in the shape of a W. Its chromatin is not so abundant as that of the lymphocyte and is located along the nuclear envelope. A Golgi complex (Go) is seen at the indented portion of the nucleus. Several mitochondria (m), a number of small dense granules (g) which may correspond to the azure granules in light microscopy, and strands of granular endoplasmic reticulum (Er) are dispersed throughout the cytoplasm. Vacuoles (Va) and cytoplasmic projections (p), presumably of pinocytotic nature, are present in the peripheral cytoplasm.

Lc : Lymphocyte.
Pl : Blood platelet.
R : Erythrocyte.

From the peripheral blood of a 36-year-old male which was fixed by 1.0% glutaraldehyde followed by 2.0% osmium tetroxide post-fixation. Stained with uranyl acetate and lead tartarate solution. ×12,000. (Photograph courtesy of Dr. A. HATTORI)

REFERENCES:

ANDERSEN, D.R.: Ultrastructure of normal and leukemic leukocytes in human peripheral blood. J. Ultrastr. Res. suppl., *9*: 1966.
BESSIG, M. and J. THIERY: Electron microscopy of human white blood cells and their stem cells. Intern. Rev. Cytol., *12*: 199–241, 1961.
INMAN, D.R. and E.H. COOPER: Electron microscopy of human lymphocytes stimulated by phytohaemagglutinin. J. Cell Biol., *19*: 441–445, 1963.
WATANABE, I., S. DONAHUE and N. HOGGATT: Method for electron microscopic studies of circulating human leukocytes and observations on their fine structure. J. Ultrastr. Res., *20*: 366–382, 1967.

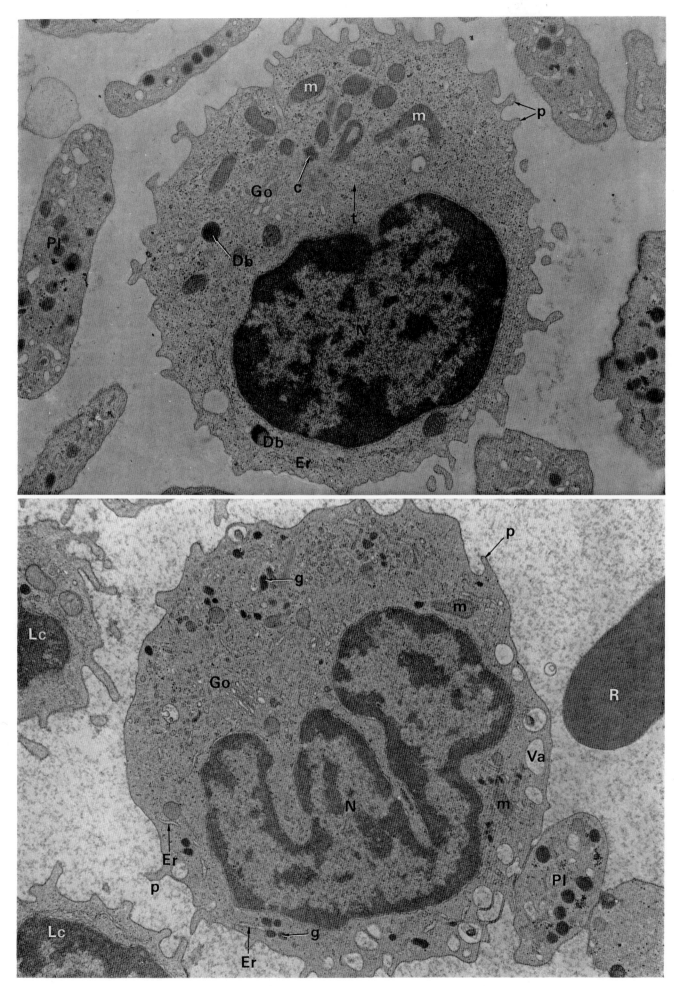

37

Neutrophilic granulocyte

The neutrophilic granulocytes occupy from 55 to 60 per cent of the total leukocyte count in peripheral blood and measure from 9 to 12 μ in diameter. They are highly amoeboid and phagocytic, and contain fine cytoplasmic granules which correspond to the neutrophilic granules in light microscopy. The nucleus is rod-like in younger forms and becomes segmented in mature cells. The segments are connected by thin strings of nuclear substance.

Top: This micrograph shows a mature neutrophilic granulocyte with a nucleus separated into four lobes (N). The nucleoplasm is largely occupied by heavily stained chromatin which is condensed beneath the nuclear envelope. Nucleoli do not occur.

The dense cytoplasm is packed with membrane-bounded granules which are, in the aldehyde-fixed cells as in this case, divided into two types: large, round, electron-dense granules (g_1) and small, round or rod-shaped, very electron-dense granules (g_2). However, there are transitions between the two types, and many granules can not definitely be identified as one or the other. In electron microscopic histochemistry, it was demonstrated that the large type granules contained peroxidase and such hydrolytic enzymes as acid phosphatase. This finding indicates that they may correspond to lysosomes which serve in the digestion of phagocytized materials. On the other hand, the small, very dense granules were found to contain large amounts of alkaline phosphatase, but their function remains obscure at present.

Besides the granules, the cytoplasm contains a few numbers of small mitochondria (m), glycogen particles and a few strands of granular endoplasmic reticulum. A centriole (c) and a small Golgi complex (Go) are seen near the center of the cell.

Peripheral blood of a 37-year-old female. Fixation with phosphate-buffered 1.0% glutaraldehyde followed by post-fixation with 2.0% osmium tetroxide solution. Stained with uranyl acetate and lead tartarate solution. ×22,000. (Photograph courtesy of Dr. A. HATTORI)

Bottom: A portion of a neutrophilic granulocyte is shown in this micrograph. The appearance of the granules conspicuously differs in this cell fixed singly in osmium from that in the case of aldehyde fixation. The granules in this micrograph vary in profile from granule to granule, but they are difficult to classify into two types by their electron density.

m: Mitochondrion.
N: Nucleus.

Peripheral blood of a 45-year-old male. Fixation with s-collidine-buffered 2.0% osmium tetroxide. Stained with lead tartarate solution. ×35,000. (Photograph courtesy of Dr. A. HATTORI)

REFERENCES:

GOODMAN, J. R., E. B. REILLY and R. E. MOORE: Electron microscopy of formed elements of normal human blood. Blood, *12*: 428–442, 1957.
HAYHOE, F. G. J. and R. J. FLEMANS: An atlas of haematological cytology. Wolfe, London, 1969.
HIRSCH, J. G. and M. E. FEDORKO: Ultrastructure of human leukocytes after simultaneous fixation with glutaraldehyde and osmium tetroxide and "postfixation" in uranyl acetate. J. Cell Biol., *38*: 615–627, 1968.
NEWSOME, J.: Phagocytosis by human neutrophils. Nature, *214*: 1092–1094, 1967.

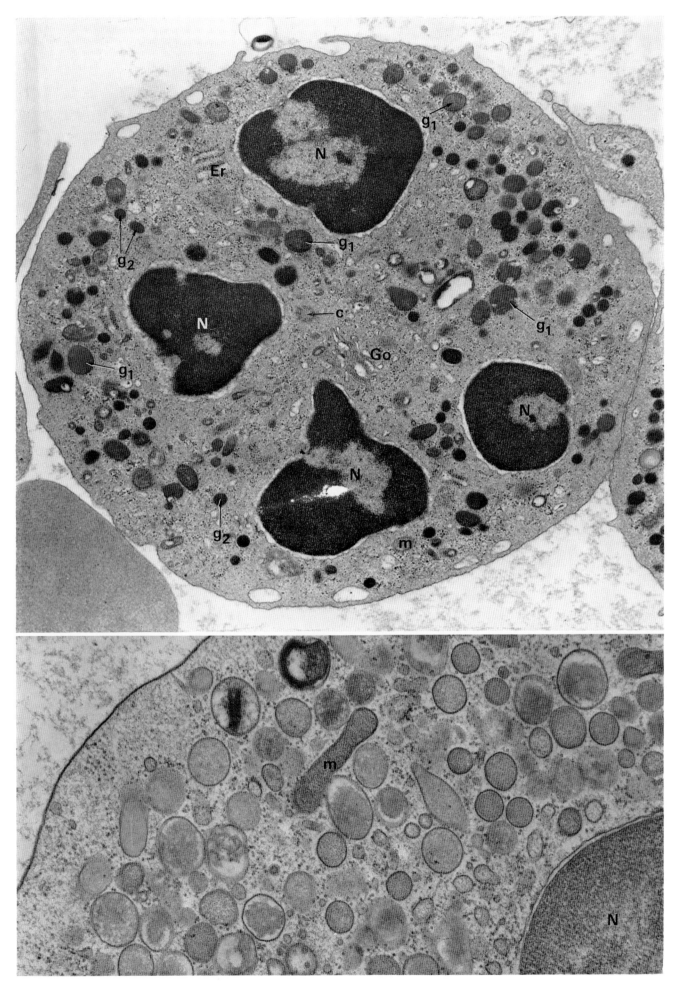

39

Eosinophilic granulocyte

Eosinophilic granulocytes comprise 3 to 5 per cent of the total leukocyte count in peripheral blood. The characteristically large eosinophilic granules in Giemsa-stained smears, are, in electron microscopy, membrane-bounded ellipsoidal bodies measuring from 0.5 to 1.0 μ in diameter. They contain a dense, plate-like core which is surrounded by a fine granular matrix of relatively low electron density. The core of the granule often shows many parallel lamellae, the periodicity of which is, in human beings, about 40Å. The core contains an abundance of phospholipids and peroxidase. In cytochemistry, the matrix of the specific granules shows positive activities in acid-phosphatase and peroxidase, indicating the lysosomal character of the eosinophilic granules.

Top: A survey view of an eosinophilic granulocyte. The nucleus is oval in shape with a prominent nucleolus (Nu). Chromatin is condensed beneath the nuclear envelope. The main part of the cytoplasm is packed with specific granules (g). Sacs of granular endoplasmic reticulum (Er) are dilated, perhaps due to osmium tetroxide fixation. Mitochondria (m) are not frequent.

Peripheral blood of a 54-year-old male with gastric ulcer. Fixed by s-collidine-buffered 2.0% osmium tetroxide. Stained with lead tartarate solution. ×14,000. (Photograph courtesy of Dr. A. Hattori)

Bottom: A portion of an eosinophilic leucocyte showing a few of its granules at high magnification. The granules are bounded by a limiting membrane and contain a crystalloid core surrounded by a fine granular material. In this picture the characteristic lamellar structure of the crystalloid plate can not be observed.

N: Nucleus.

Bone marrow of a 15-year-old female with subsepsis allergica. Fixed by 1.0% glutaraldehyde and then post-fixed with 2.0% osmium tetroxide solution in phosphate buffer. Stained with uranyl acetate and lead tartarate solution. ×48,000.

REFERENCES:

Faller, A.: Zur Frage von Struktur und Aufbau der eosinophilen Granula. Z. Zellforsch., *69*: 551–565, 1966.

Miller, F., E. de Harven and G. E. Palade: The structure of eosinophil leukocyte granules in rodents and in man. J. Cell Biol., *31*: 349–362, 1966.

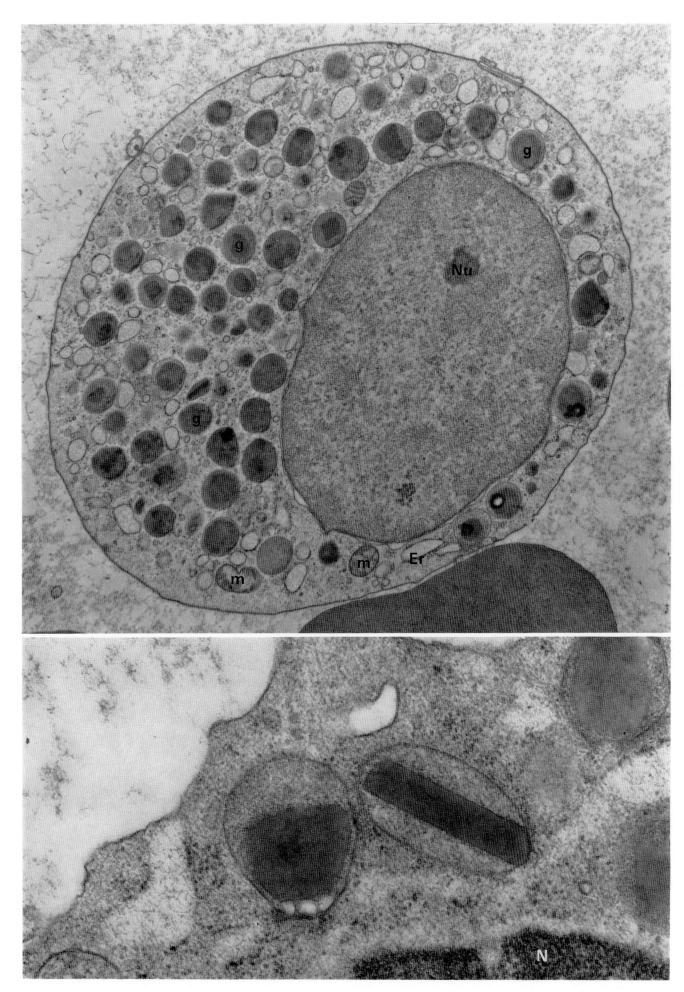

41

Basophilic granulocyte

Basophilic granulocytes, which are from 10 to 12 μ in diameter, are the cells of lowest frequency in normal peripheral blood, being about 0.5 per cent of the total leukocyte count. In Giemsa stained smears, they are characterized by the presence of large basophilic granules (g) which are soluble in water. These granules are metachromatic and contain, like mast cell granules, large amounts of heparin and histamine. They are, in electron microscopy, membrane-bounded bodies measuring from 0.4 to 1.0 μ in diameter. Usually they are tightly packed with fine particles of hgih electron density. They may, however, appear homogeneous or vacuolar.

The nucleus (N) of the basophilic granulocyte is not segmented and lacks a nucleolus. The chromatin network is not so dense as the neutrophilic granulocyte. Cisterns of granular endoplasmic reticulum (Er) and mitochondria (m) are seen among the specific granules. A few glycogen particles (Gl) are scattered throughout the cytoplasm.

Top: A basophilic granulocyte seen in peripheral blood. The cell surface extrudes to form irregular cytoplasmic processes (p). The nucleus (N) is U-shaped.

Bottom: A portion of a basophilic granulocyte showing the detail of the specific granules.

Go: Golgi complex.

Top and Bottom: From the peripheral blood of 36-year-old male. Fixed by 1.0% glutaraldehyde and then by 2.0% osmium tetroxide solution in phosphate buffer. Stained with uranyl acetate and lead tartarate solution. Top: ×15,000. Bottom: ×38,000. (Photographs courtesy of Dr. A. HATTORI)

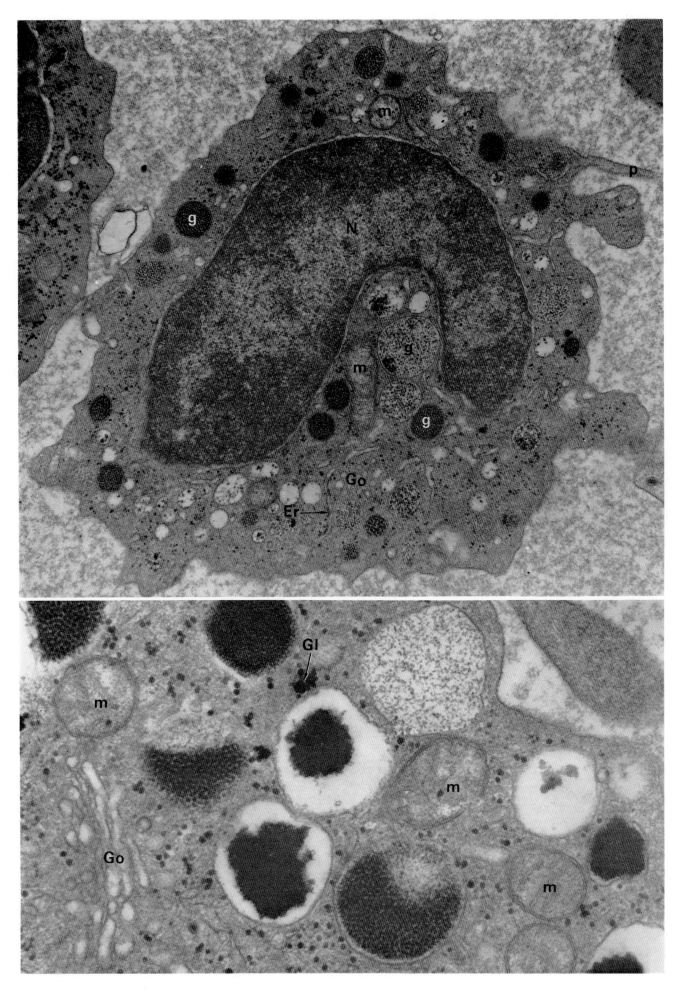

43

Blood platelet and fibrin strand

The blood platelets are small, separated portions of the cytoplasm of the megakaryocyte. By releasing platelet factors, they play an essential role in blood coagulation.

The blood platelet is a lens-like disc consisting of two parts: a peripheral clear area called hyalomere and a central granular area called granulomere. The hyalomere is characterized by the presence of bundles of microtubules with a central core (t) running circularly beneath the plasma membrane and channels opening to the surface, giving a spongy appearance to the blood platelet (arrows). Microtubules are thought to be responsible for maintaining the lens-like shape of the blood platelet. The granulomere contains several round or oval granules (g) which vary in electron density. They contain hydrolytic enzymes such as acid phosphatase and may be lysosomes. Small mitochondria (m) with a few cristae, glycogen particles (Gl) and some vesicles (v) and vacuoles (Va) are also contained in the granulomere.

The blood platelets produce thromboplastin which is involved in the transformation of liver-born prothrombin into thrombin. In coagulation of blood, the action of thrombin forms fibrin strands from fibrinogen. Under the electron microscope, they show a characteristic crossbanding which is repeated at intervals of about 240Å. A thin sub-band is seen within each 240Å period.

Ts: Tubular system.

Top: A perpendicular section of a blood platelet.
Middle left: A cross section of a blood platelet.
Middle right: A marginal portion of a blood platelet shown in higher magnification. Note central cores of microtubules.

Peripheral blood of a 31-year-old male. Fixation with phosphate-buffered 1.0% glutaraldehyde followed by post-fixation with 1.0% osmium tetroxide solution. Stained with uranyl acetate and lead tartarate. Top: ×38,000. Middle left: ×25,000. Middle right: ×57,000. (Photographs courtesy of Dr. A. Hattori)

Bottom: Fibrin strand showing the periodic cross striation.

Peripheral blood of a 34-year-old male. Fixed with s-collidine-buffered osmium tetroxide. Stained with lead tartarate. ×100,000. (Photograph courtesy of Dr. A. Hattori)

REFERENCES:

Behnke, O.: Further studies on microtubles. A marginal bundle in human and rat thrombocytes. J. Ultrastr. Res., *13*: 469–477, 1965.

Hattori, A.: Electron microscopy of human blood platelets (in Japanese). Blood and Vessel (Japan), *1*: 667–703, 1970.

Hovig, T.: The ultrastructure of blood platelets in normal and abnormal states. In: K. G. Jensen and S. Killmann (ed.): Blood Platelets (Series haematologica. vol. I-2. p. 3-64), Munksgaard, Copenhagen, 1968.

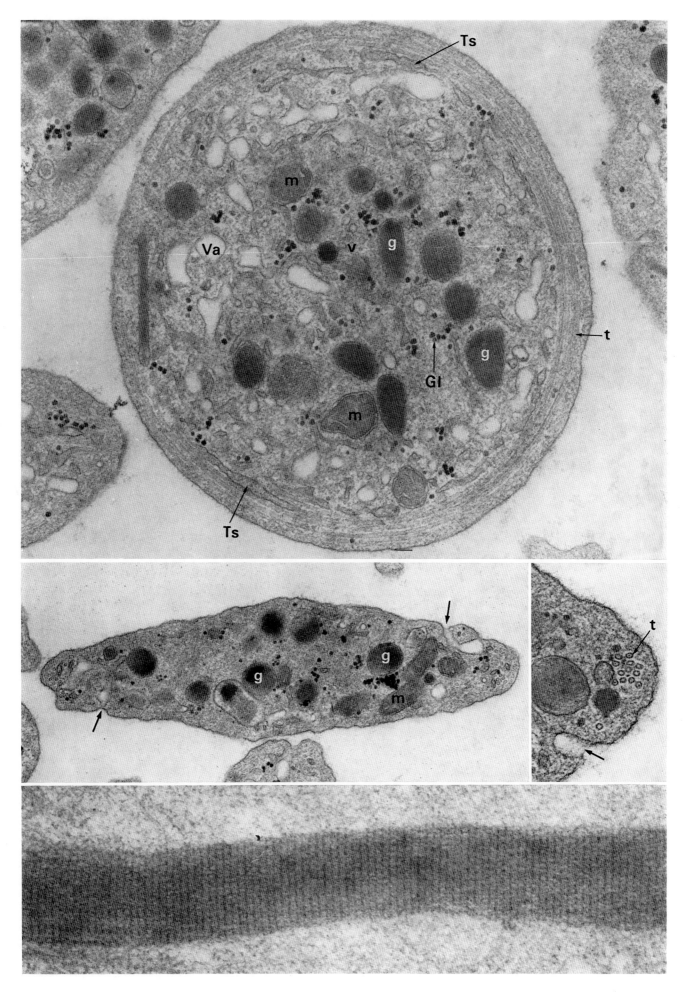

45

BLOOD AND BONE MARROW

Myeloblast and reticular cell

The framework of bone marrow is formed by reticular cells associated with reticular fibers. Various hematopoietic cells and fat cells occupy the interstices of the framework. The reticular cells have a phagocytotic property and are thought to retain the developmental potentialities of primitive mesenchymal cells.

This micrograph shows two myeloblasts (Mbl), a reticular cell (Rc) and partial profiles of other cells such as mature neutrophilic granulocytes (Nl) and plasma cells (Pc).

The nucleus of the myeloblast is large and slightly deformed and has prominent nucleoli (Nu). The karyoplasm is relatively homogeneous. The condensation of chromatin is not conspicuous. The cytoplasm shows abundant free ribosomes, several cisterns of granular endoplasmic reticulum (Er), a small Golgi complex (Go) and some mitochondria (m). A small number of specific granules (g) is seen, especially in the periphery of the cell. Some of them have a clear zone beneath the limiting membrane (arrows).

The reticular cell is characterized by an irregular contour with long cytoplasmic processes. In the cytoplasm are seen a centriole (c), several lysosomes (Ly), mitochondria (m), strands of granular endoplasmic reticulum (Er) and Golgi complexes (Go).

Bone marrow of a 15-year-old female with subsepsis allergica. Phosphate-buffered 2.5% glutaraldehyde fixation followed by post-fixation with 2.0% osmium tetroxide solution. Uranyl acetate and lead tartarate staining. ×7,300.

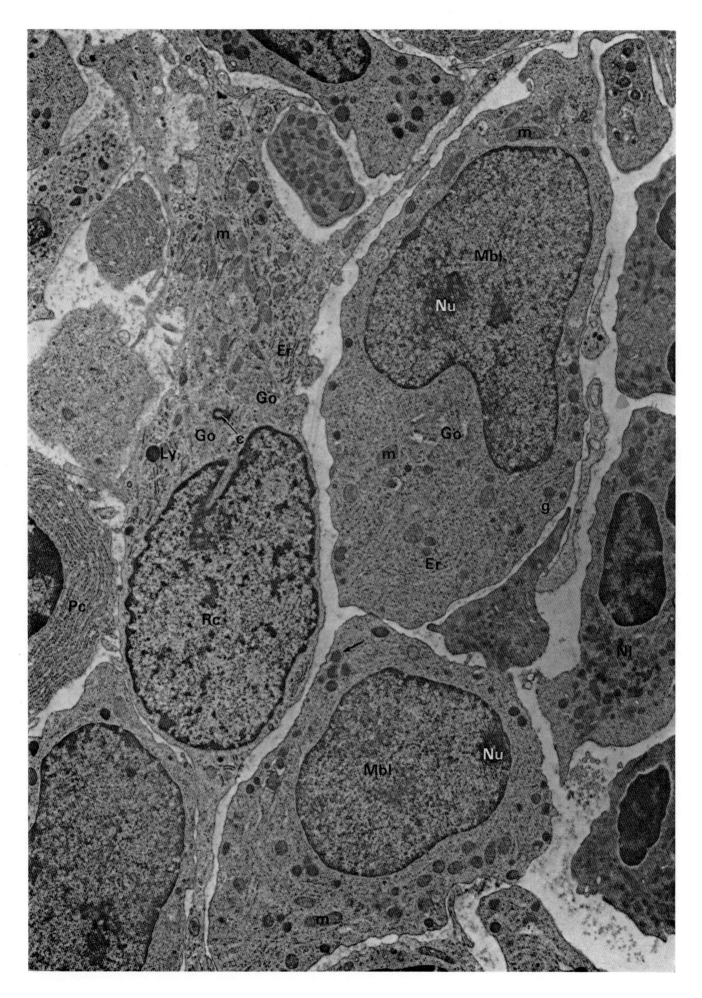

47

Proerythroblast and erythroblast

The proerythroblast (Pre) is the earliest recognizable stage in the differentiation of an erythrocyte. As shown in this picture, it is large in size and has a round, clear nucleus with a prominent nucleolus (Nu). The cytoplasm is clear and contains a centriole (c), Golgi complexes (Go), abundant free ribosomes in the form of polysomes, mitochondria (m), a few strands of granular endoplasmic reticulum, several dense bodies and bundles of microtubular structures (∗).

In the course of the development of the proerythroblast, the chromatin of the nucleus becomes condensed and the cytoplasm increases in density, due mainly to the accumulation of hemoglobin; this leads to the differentiation of the erythroblast.

This picture contains several profiles of erythroblasts (Erb). As compared with the proerythroblast, their cytoplasm and nucleus appear darker and their mitochondria are somewhat smaller. Centrioles (c) and Golgi complexes (Go) are also found. Coated vesicles suggesting the pinocytotic activity of the cell are seen beneath the surface of the cell (arrows).

Lym :   Lymphocyte.
R :   Mature erythrocyte.
Rc :   Reticular cell.

Bone marrow of a 21-year-old female in complete remission from aplastic anemia. Fixed in phosphate-buffered 1.0% glutaraldehyde and then post-fixed with 2.0% osmium tetroxide. Stained with uranyl acetate and lead tartarate solution. ×11,000. (Photograph courtesy of Dr. A. HATTORI)

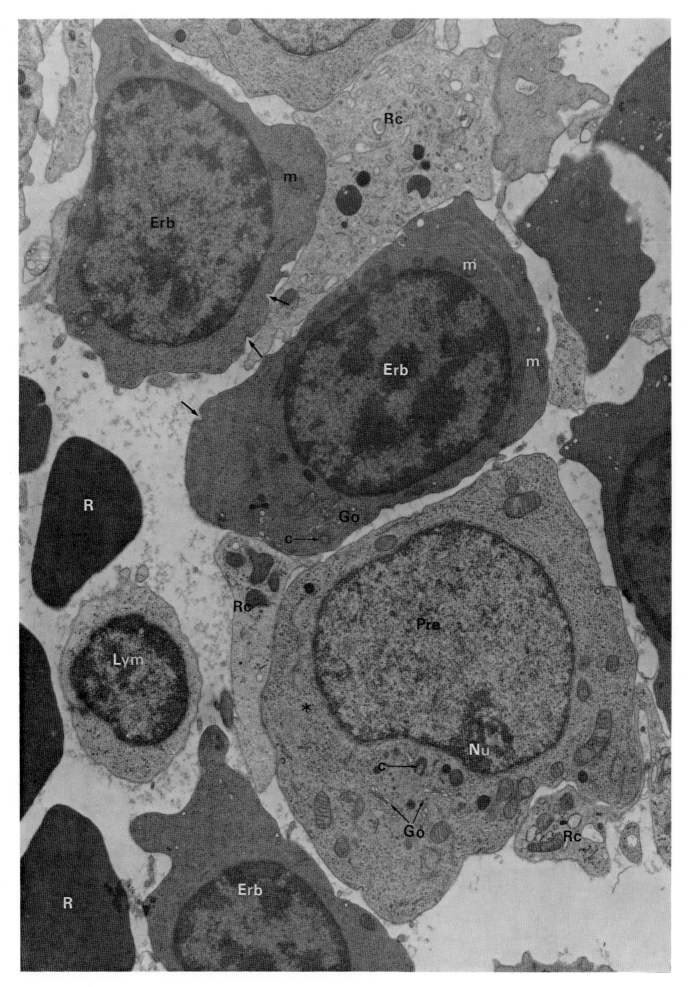

49

Granulopoietic cells in the bone marrow

In the normal adult, the source of granular leukocytes is the bone marrow. This picture shows a portion of bone marrow containing neutrophilic granulocytes in different stages of maturation: myeloblast (Mbl), promyelocyte (Pro), myelocyte (My), metamyelocyte (Mt) and mature neutrophilic granulocytes (Nl). Collectively, these cells are termed granulopoietic cells. The myeloblast, promyelocyte and myelocyte increase in number by cell-divisions, but in the metamyelocyte and mature granulocyte no further cell-division occurs.

The myeloblast is the earliest recognizable cell in the differentiation of granulopoietic cells. It has a large, clear nucleus with irregular indentations and prominent nucleoli. Its cytoplasm contains free ribosomes, strands of granular endoplasmic reticulum and mitochondria. A small number of cytoplasmic granules is found.

The promyelocyte is the largest in the granulopoietic cells. The nucleus is large and the chromatin is slightly clumped along the nuclear envelope. The cytoplasm is very rich, and contains well-developed cisterns of granular endoplasmic reticulum, prominent Golgi complexes and numerous cytoplasmic granules. The myelocyte is characterized by a number of large, round, cytoplasmic granules. It also contains small, very dense granules. The latter increase in number with the maturation of the cell. The metamyelocyte has a kidney-shaped nucleus with chromatin clumped along the nuclear envelope. With the maturation of the cell, its cytoplasm becomes increasingly dense and the chromatin of the nucleus more and more condensed. The mature neutrophilic granulocyte has a nucleus with condensed chromatin and dark cytoplasm packed with numerous cytoplasmic granules of various sizes and shapes.

Material and method are the same as those of the picture on page 49. ×6,000. (Photograph courtesy of Dr. A. HATTORI)

REFERENCE:

SCOTT, R. E.: Ultrastructural aspects of neutrophil granulocyte development in humans. Lab. Invest., *23*: 202-215, 1970.

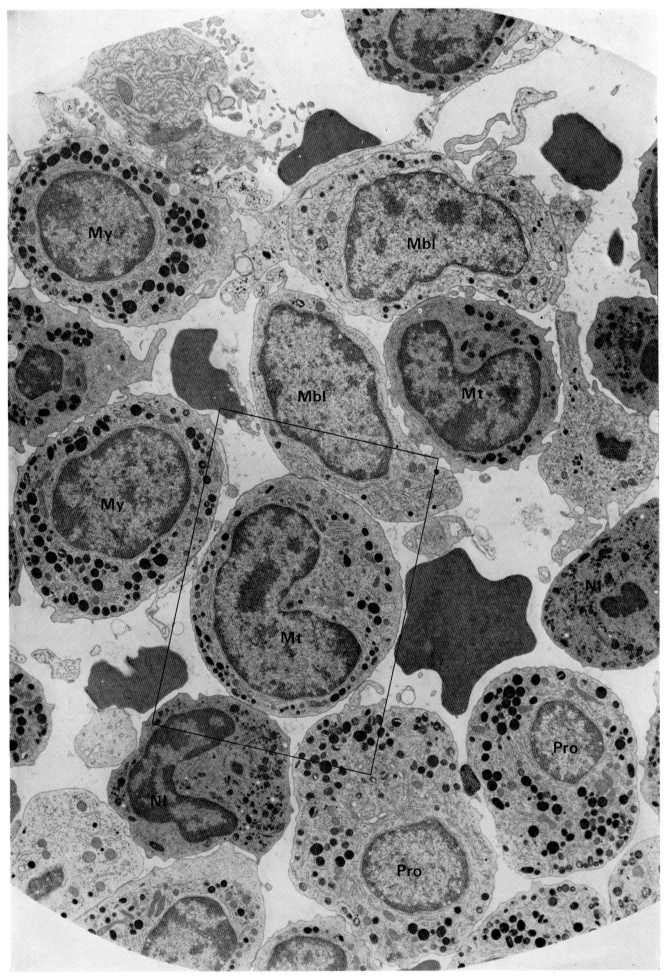

51

Promyelocyte (Top)

The promyelocyte shown in this picture has a large, round nucleus with two prominent nucleoli (Nu). The chromatin is relatively evenly dispersed in the nucleoplasm and its condensation beneath the nuclear envelope is not conspicuous. The cytoplasm is characterized by dilated cisterns of granular endoplasmic reticulum (Er), well-developed Golgi complexes (Go) which are located on one side of the nucleus, and cytoplasmic granules (g) of different density and internal structure. The surface of the cell is relatively smooth.

m : Mitochondrion.

Neutrophilic metamyelocyte (Bottom)

This picture is a close view of the small area enclosed in the box on the picture on page 51. The metamyelocyte shown in this picture has a kidney-shaped nucleus. Chromatin is condensed beneath the nuclear envelope. Golgi complexes (Go) are near the indentation of the nucleus. Besides large, dense granules (g_1), finer granules (g_2) have appeared. The large granules are two to three times more numerous than the small ones. Small quantities of ribosomes and granular endoplasmic reticulum are seen in the cytoplasm.

Top and Bottom: Material and method are the same as those of the picture on page 49. Top: ×11,000. Bottom: ×13,000. (Photographs courtesy of Dr. A. HATTORI)

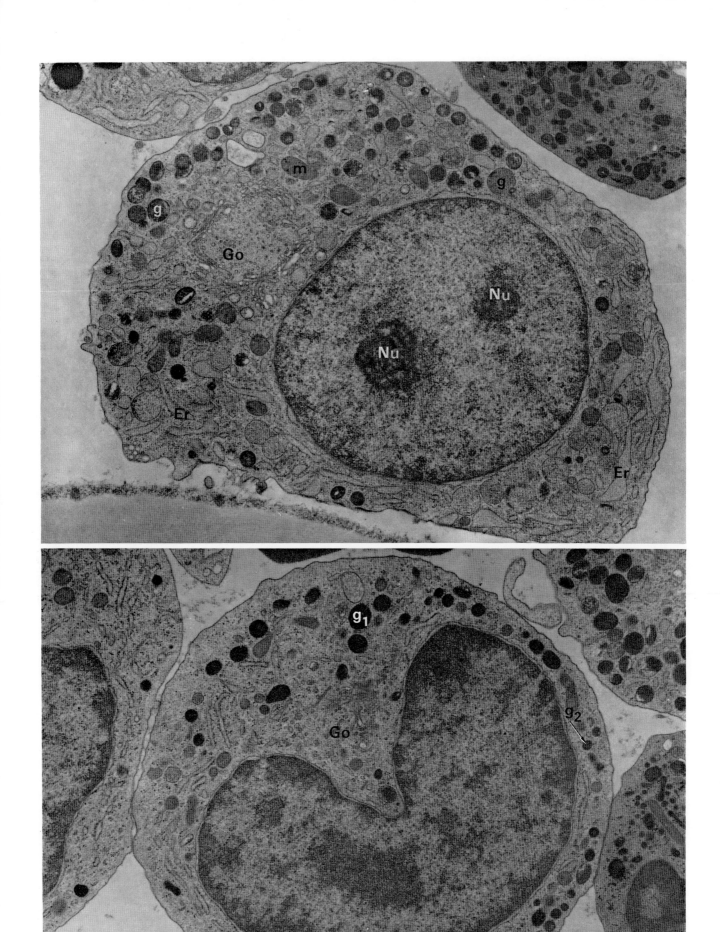

53

Megakaryocyte

The megakaryocyte, the mother cell of blood platelets, is a giant cell of the bone marrow. The nucleus of a mature megakaryocyte is separated into several lobes which are connected by strands of nuclear material. The nucleoplasm is characterized by the presence of multiple small nucleoli (Nu). The cytoplasm is very rich and is divided into three zones from the nucleus to the margin: endoplasm, intermediate zone and ectoplasm. The endoplasm (En) is the zone surrounded by the lobes of the nucleus. It contains centrioles, Golgi complexes, abundant membrane-bound granules (g), ribosomes and some glycogen particles. The intermediate zone (Iz) is the wide zone between the nucleus and the plasma membrane. This zone is characterized by the presence of a large communicating system of flattened cisterns. Small regions of the cytoplasm, which become blood platelets in future, are almost completely limited by a smooth-surfaced membrane. The latter becomes the plasma membrane of the blood platelets and is called platelet demarcation membrane (Pdm). The ectoplasm (Ec) is the outer cytoplasm, appearing relatively homogeneous with few cell organelles. In mature megakaryocytes, the intermediate zone is so voluminous that the other zones may sometimes be not noticeable.

Fc : Fat cell.
L : Lymphocyte.
N : Nucleus.
Nl : Neutrophilic leukocyte.

Top : A survey picture of a mature megakaryocyte.
Bottom : A portion of a megakaryocyte.

Top and Bottom : Material and method are the same as those of the picture on page 47. Top : ×4,600. Bottom : ×19,000.

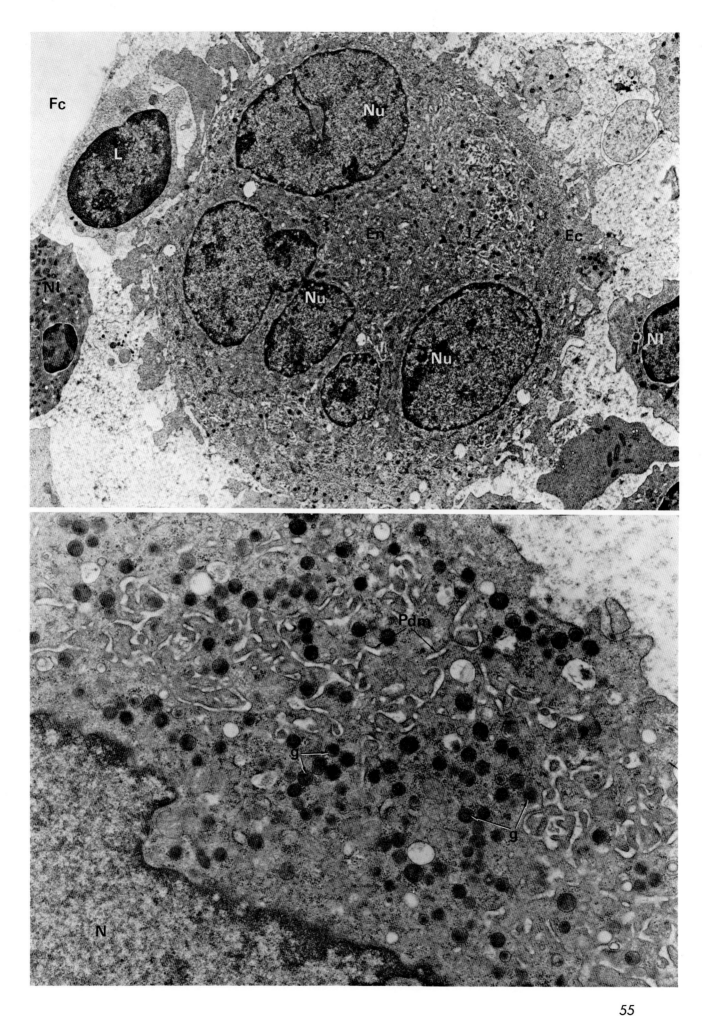

55

Germinal center of the lymphatic follicle

In the cortical follicle of the lymph node, the central portion, in which lymphocytes are actively produced, is called the germinal center. In this micrograph there are large, round, lymphatic cells. These cells are called lymphogonia or hemocytoblasts (Hb) and are considered the most primitive stage of lymphatic cells. They are characterized by a large nucleus (N) with prominent nucleoli (Nu), by an abundance of free ribosomes in a narrow cytoplasm and by the large mitochondria (m) with clear matrix. The mitotic cell (Mi) seen in the lower right corner of this micrograph is presumably a lymphoblast.

Go: Golgi complex.
Lb: Lymphoblast.
Mp: Macrophage.
Prc: Cytoplasmic process of reticular cell.

Mesenterial lymph node of a 61-year-old male patient of esophageal cancer. Obtained by surgical operation. Fixation in 2.0% glutaraldehyde followed by 2.0% osmium tetroxide in phosphate buffer. Uranyl acetate and lead tartarate staining. ×7,000.

REFERENCES:

BERNHARD, W. and R. LEPLUS: Fine structure of the normal and malignant human lymph node. Pergamon Press, Oxford, 1964.

BROOKS, R. E. and B. V. SIEGEL: Normal human lymph node cells: An electron microscopic study. Blood, *27*: 687–705, 1966.

MORI, Y. and K. LENNERT: Electron microscopic atlas of lymph node cytology and pathology. Springer-Verlag, Berlin, 1969.

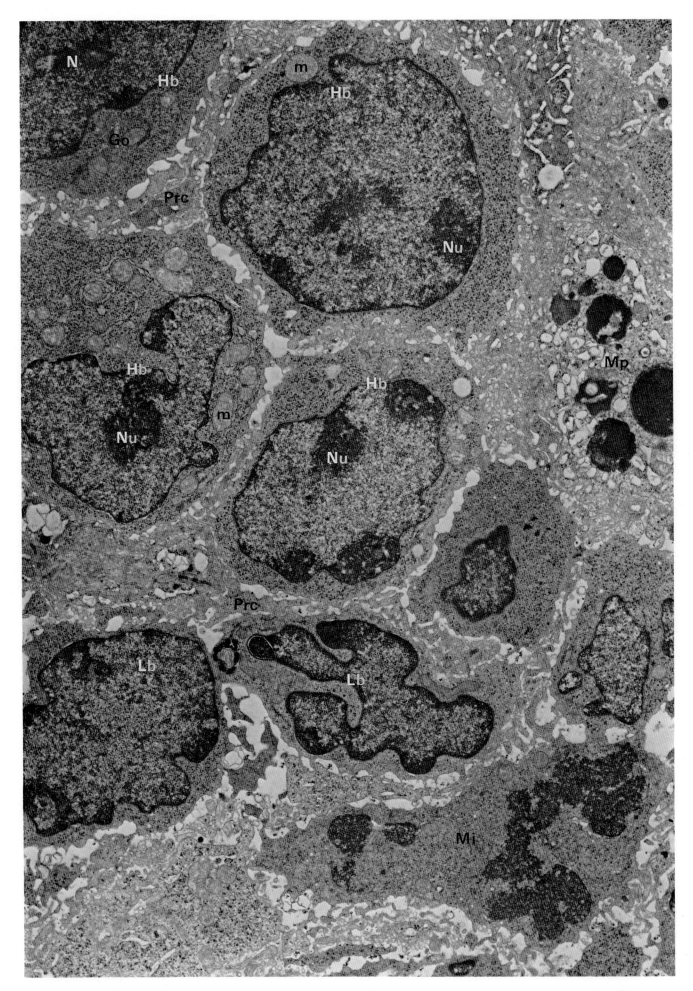

57

LYMPH NODE

Lymphoblast (Top)

The lymphoblast is a premature lymphocyte and increases in number by cell division as shown in the picture on page 57. This micrograph is from the peripheral zone of a cortical follicle. The lymphoblast has an irregularly-shaped nucleus (N) with abundant chromatin (Ch) in its periphery. Mitochondria (m), which are smaller in size and higher in density than those of hemocytoblasts, tend to gather on one side of the cell. Free ribosomes are relatively abundant. A Golgi complex (Go) and centrioles (c) are present in the indentation of the nucleus (N).

        Pc: Plasma cell.
        Rc: Reticular cell.

Lymphatic sinus (Bottom)

This micrograph shows a lymphatic sinus seen in the cortical zone of a lymph node. The sinus is lined by flattened sinal endothelial cells (Sed) which are thought to belong to the reticuloendothelial system. The nucleus (N) is similar in its chromatin pattern to that of the reticular cell (Rc) seen in the adjacent parenchyme. The cytoplasm contains several dense bodies (Db). Besides lymphocytes (Lc), a neutrophilic leucocyte (Nl) is seen within the sinal lumen (Slu). The basal lamina (Bl) underlying the sinal endothelial cells is not continuous (arrow).

Top and Bottom: Material and method are the same as those of the picture on page 57. Top: ×10,000. Bottom: ×5,000.

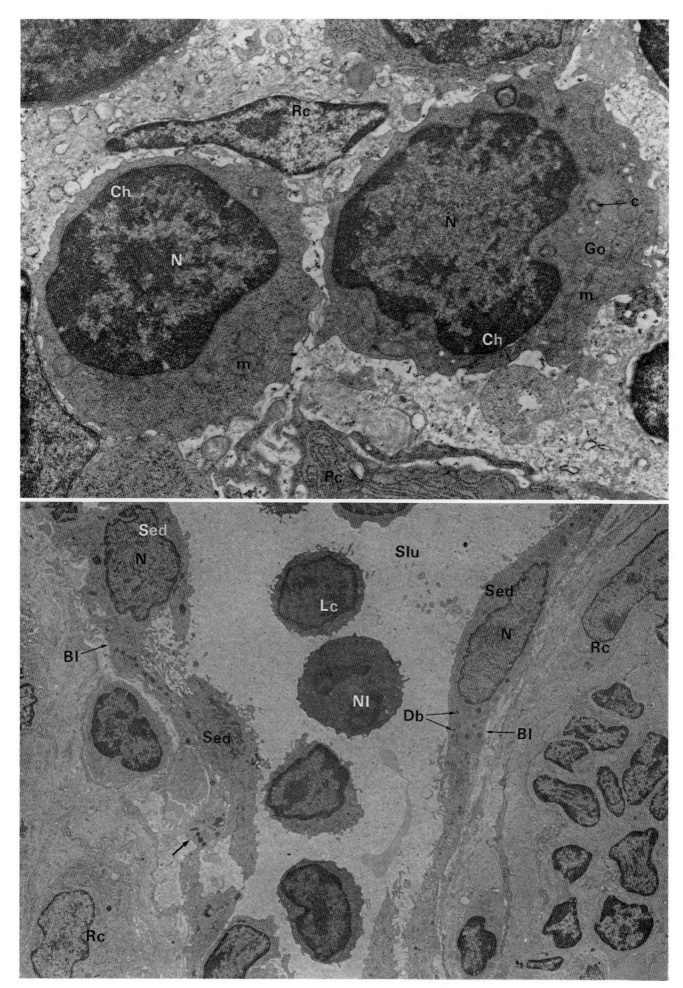

Cortex of the thymus

The thymus is a lymphoid organ which, in fetal and infantile life, produces antibody-making cells: lymphocytes and plasma cells. The cells originated from the thymus are then delivered to various sites of the whole body where they colonize to form the lymph nodes and nodules, tonsils and other lymphatic tissues.

Histologically, the thymus consists of a number of lobules which are divided into cortex and medulla. The framework of both cortex and medulla is formed by a spongy meshwork of epithelial reticular cells and a parenchyme consisting of lymphocytes, often called thymocytes, and macrophages called mesenchymal reticular cells. In the cortex, the lymphocytes are far more numerous than the reticular cells. The medulla consists mainly of reticular cells and contains characteristic Hassal's bodies or thymic corpuscles.

This is a low-power electron micrograph showing a portion of the cortex of the thymus. The majority of the cells (Tc) are lymphocytes. The cells with large, pale nuclei are epithelial reticular cells (Rc) forming a meshwork throughout the thymus.

From the thymus of a 7-month fetus ($\female$, 800 g). Phosphate-buffered 2.5% glutaraldehyde fixation followed by 1.3% osmium tetroxide post-fixation. Uranyl acetate and lead tartarate staining. ×5,500.

REFERENCES:

HIROKAWA, K.: Electron microscopic observation of the human thymus of the fetus and the new born. Acta pathol. jap., *19*: 1-13, 1969.

ITO, T., T. HOSHINO and K. ABE: The fine structure of myoid cells in the human thymus. Arch. histol. jap., *30*: 207-215, 1969.

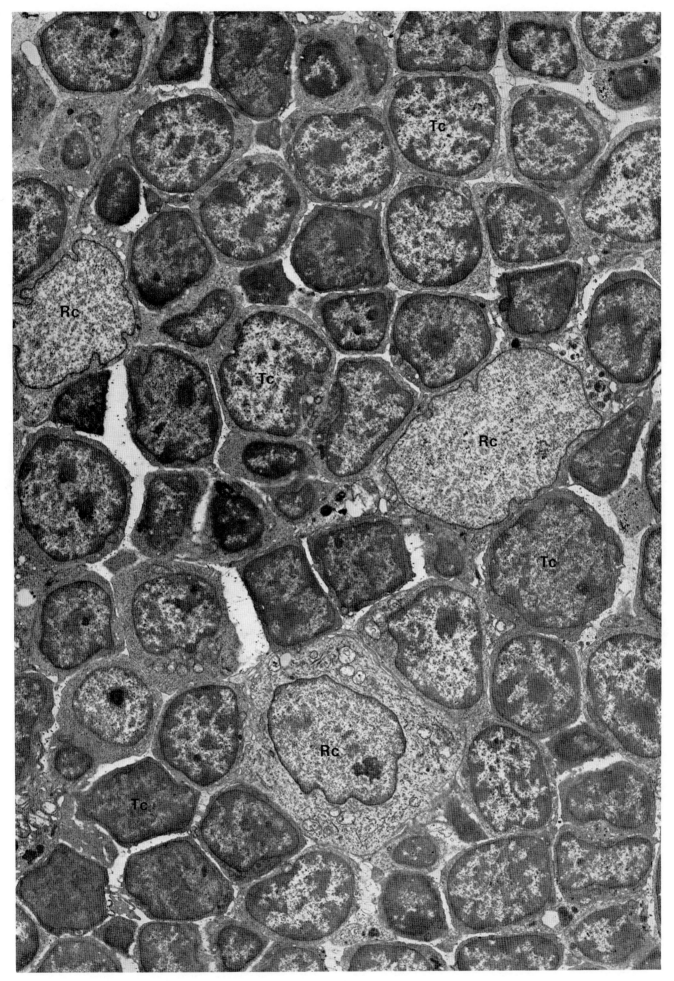

61

Hassall's corpuscle

Hassall's corpuscles are small bodies characteristically found in the medulla of the thymus. They vary from 20 to more than 100 μ in diameter and are composed of concentrically-arranged, flattened cells. Central portions of them often show features of degeneration. It is said that the Hassall's body originates from endodermal reticular cells.

N :   Nucleus.
Rc: Reticular cell.

Thymus of a 6-month fetus (♂, 600 g). Phosphate-buffered 2.5% glutaraldehyde fixation followed by 2.0% osmium tetroxide post-fixation. Uranyl acetate and lead tartarate staining. ×6,000. (Photograph courtesy of Dr. Y. Matsukura)

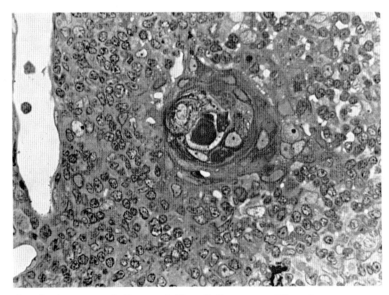

A light micrograph of an area of the medulla of thymus: The thymocytes are not so numerous in the medulla as in the cortex, and the reticular cells with large, pale nuclei are prominent and predominant. The profile of a blood capillary in the upper left corner contains two lymphocytes. A Hassall's corpuscle is seen in the center of this micrograph.

7-month fetus (♀, 800 g). Epon-embedded section stained with toluidine blue. ×600. (Photograph courtesy of Dr. Y. Matsukura)

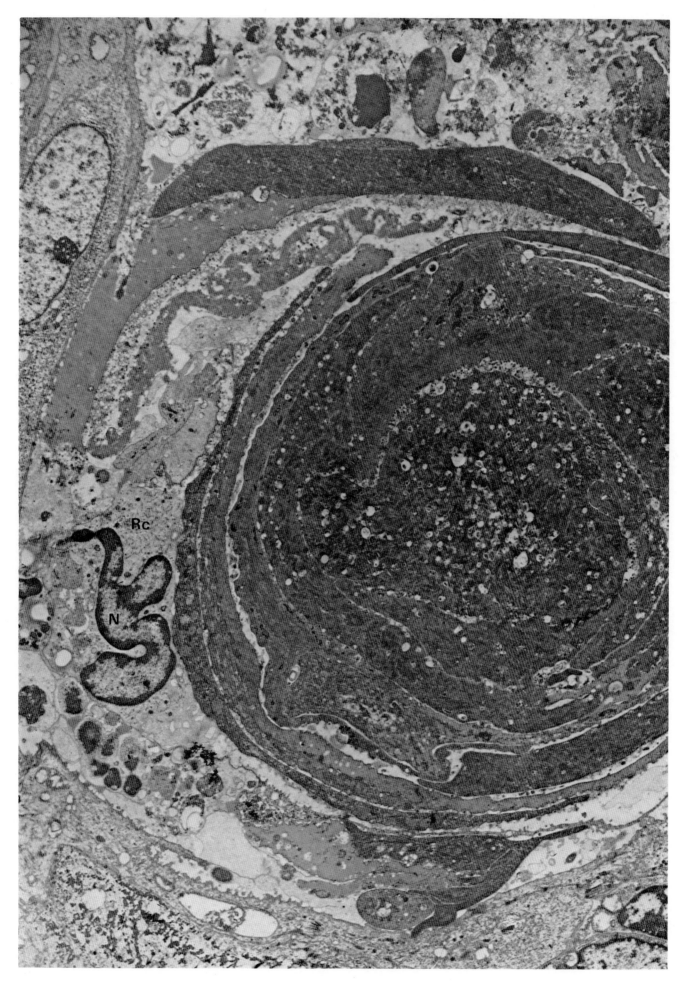

SPLEEN

Red pulp of the spleen (Top)

The red pulp of the spleen is composed of splenic sinuses and splenic cords. The sinuses are long and tortuous vascular channels lined by sinal endothelial cells (Sed) belonging to the reticuloendothelial system. The sinal basement membrane (Bm) running beneath the endothelial cells is discontinuous and varies in thickness because of the plane of the section. Within the sinal lumen, red blood cells (R), lymphocytes (Lc) and neutrophilic leukocytes (Nl) are seen. The splenic cords are spongy tissue lying among the sinuses. They are basically made of reticular cells (Rc) with long cytoplasmic processes and reticular fibers (Rf) which compose a network structure. In the meshes of these elements many cellular elements, including macrophages (Mp), red blood cells, lymphocytes and others, are packed.

Sinal endothelial cell (Bottom)

The sinal endothelial cells are elongate cells lying parallel to the long axis of the sinal vessel and they appear cuboidal or cylindrical in cross sections. The nucleus (N) is located toward the sinal lumen (Slu), and cell organelles such as Golgi complexes (Go) and mitochondria (m) are usually present in the basal cytoplasm. Attachment structures, such as desmosomes or tight junctions, can not be seen between the adjacent cells. The thin, irregular sinal basement membrane (Bm) is thickened at places into thick reticular fibers (Rf) which are known as ring fibers in light microscopy.

    Lc : Lymphocyte.
    Prc : Process of reticular cell.
    Rc : Reticular cell.

Top and Bottom: Spleen of a 27-year-old female suffering from splenic cyst. A portion macroscopically normal was taken in surgical operation. Fixation with 2.0% glutaraldehyde followed by 2.0% osmium tetroxide post fixation in phosphate buffer. Uranyl acetate and lead tartarate staining. Top: ×2,500. Bottom: ×7,500.

REFERENCE :

HIRASAWA, Y. and H. TOKUHIRO: Electron microscopic studies on the normal spleen: Especially on the red pulp and the reticulo-endothelial cells. Blood, *35*: 201-212, 1970.

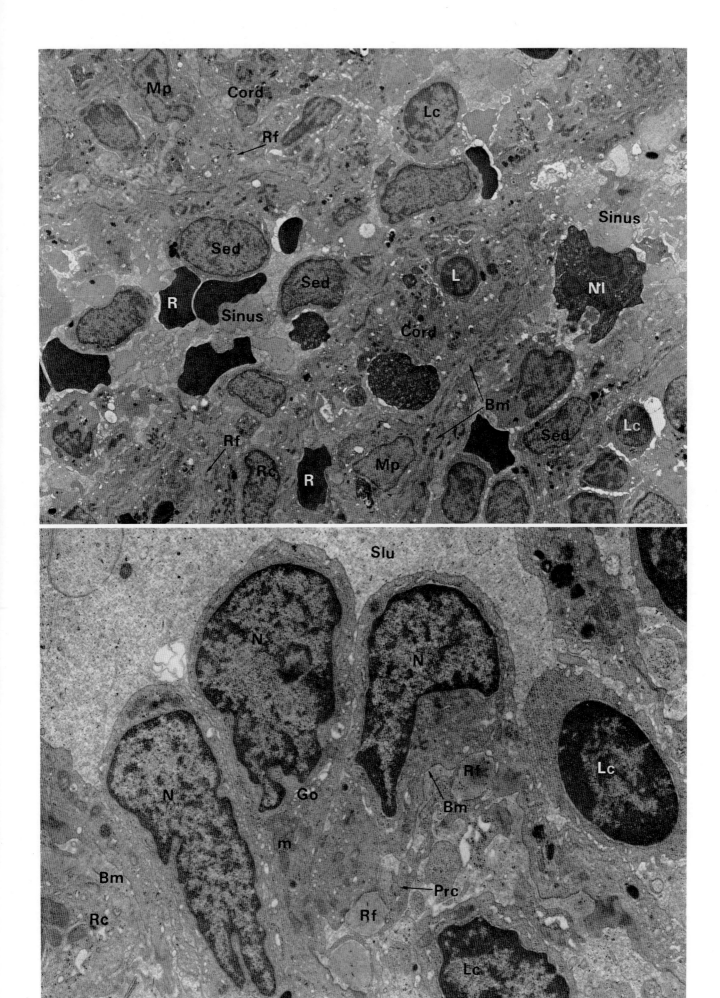

Longitudinal section of a sinal endothelial cell (Top)

When sectioned longitudinally, the lining endothelial cell shows an elongate form with tapered ends. The nucleus (N) is also elongate with many indentations. Numerous vesicles (v), possibly of micropinocytotic nature, are present in the peripheral cytoplasm. A few dense bodies (Db), numerous fine filaments (f) and free ribosomes are contained in the cytoplasm. The sinal basement membrane (Bm) runs discontinuously beneath the endothelial cell. The cytoplasmic process of a macrophage (Pmp), which seems to be passing through a gap of the basement membrane, is in contact with the cell base of the endothelial cell.

Lc :   Lymphocyte.
Mp :   Macrophage.
R :   Erythrocyte.
Rf :   Reticular fiber.
Slu :   Sinal lumen.

Erythrophagocytosis by a sinal endothelial cell (Bottom)

In the spleen, old red blood cells are phagocytized by splenic macrophages. As shown in this micrograph, a sinal endothelial cell (Scd) phagocytizing a red blood cell (R) was occasionally found in this material, though this probably reflects an unusually elevated activity of the sinal endothelial cells in this patient. A macrophage (Mp) extends its cytoplasmic process (Pr) into the sinal lumen (Slu) through the space between the endothelial cells.

Bm :   Sinal basement membrane.
Rc :   Reticular cell.
Rf :   Reticular fiber.

Top and Bottom : Material and method are the same as those of the pictures on page 65. Top: ×7,500. Bottom: ×8,500.

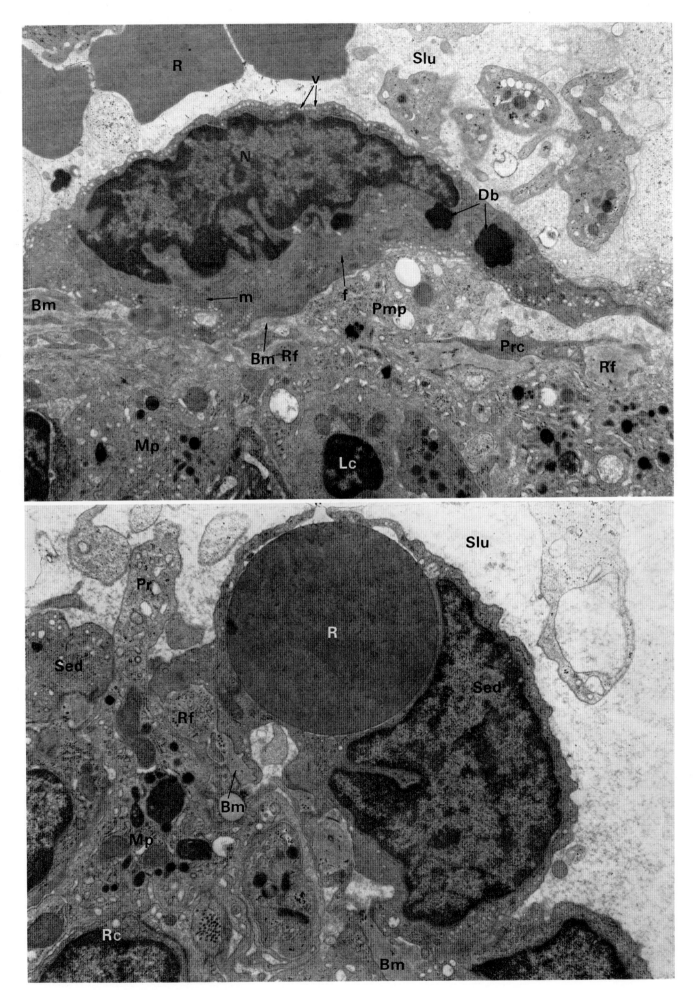

MUSCULAR TISSUE

Skeletal muscle

The basic structure of the skeletal muscle is the skeletal muscle fiber or cell. It is a long thick syncytium which arises from the fusion of the growing myoblasts. Every skeletal muscle fiber receives specialized motor nerve endings through which its contraction is mediated.

The surface of the skeletal muscle fiber is surrounded by a plasma membrane called sarcolemma with a very thick coating of polysaccharide-protein. Numerous nuclei lie immediately beneath the sarcolemma. The major part of the cytoplasm is occupied by contractile elements or myofibrils which show a characteristic cross striation. Between the myofibrils there are cell organelles such as mitochondria and specialized types of endoplasmic reticulum.

This electron micrograph shows a longitudinal section of a portion of a skeletal muscle fiber. Myofibrils show their characteristic pattern of crossbanding with A-, I-, M- and Z-bands. In the clefts between myofibrils are abundant glycogen particles, lipid droplets (Ld) and sarcoplasmic reticulum. Profiles of mitochondria (m), two to each sarcomere, occur at the I-band level. At the level where the A- and the I-bands meet, triads are located (arrows). The triad is formed by a transverse tubule which is a direct continuation of the sarcolemma and by a pair of sacs of sarcoplasmic reticulum sandwiching the former. These membrane systems mediate the transmission of excitatory nerve impulses to myofibrils.

Sa : Sarcomere.

Surgically-obtained M. tibialis anterior of a 58-year-old female. Phosphate-buffered 2.5% glutaraldehyde fixation followed by 1.0% osmium tetroxide post-fixation. Uranyl acetate and lead tartarate staining. ×19,000.

REFERENCE:

FISHER, E. R., R. E. COHN and T. S. DANOWSKI: Ultrastructural observations of skeletal muscle in myopathy and neuropathy with special reference to muscular dystrophy. Lab. Invest., *15*: 778–793, 1966.

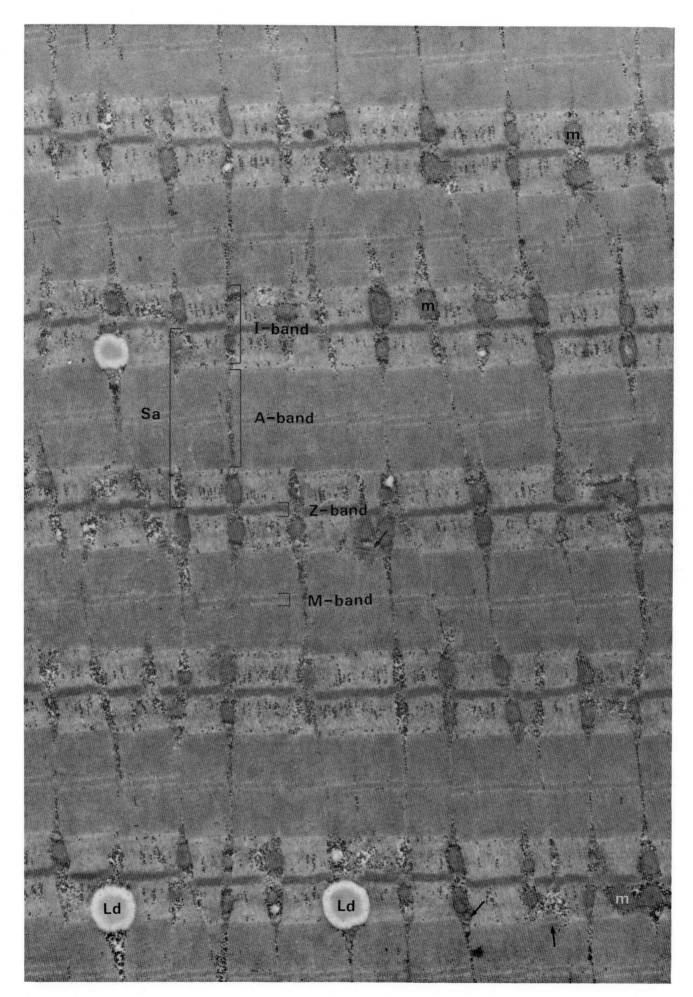

69

MUSCULAR TISSUE

Sarcomere and sarcoplasmic reticulum

Top: The sarcomere is the section of the myofibrils between two adjacent Z-bands. It is a morphological as well as a functional unit of the myofibrils.

In this picture is shown a portion of a skeletal muscle fiber containing several sarcomeres with a characteristic pattern of crossbanding. The A-band (A), the broad dark band in the sarcomere, contains thick filaments of myosin. The narrow dark stripe in the middle of the A-band is the M-band (M). The I-band (I), the broad light region between successive A-bands, is divided into two parts by the dense Z-band (Z). The thin actin filaments extend from the Z-band, through the I-band, to the beginning of the H-band, the light zone within the A-band which is not clearly seen in this picture.

When the muscle fiber contracts, the length of the A-band remains constant but that of the H- and I-band varies. It is thought that the thick and the thin filaments of the sarcomere slide back and forth; *i.e.*, the length of the filaments remains the same, but their degree of interdigitation varies.

This picture further shows profiles of the sarcoplasmic reticulum, a special network formed around the sarcomere. At the M-band level the sac of sarcoplasmic reticulum is penetrated by numerous small pores or fenestrations (arrows). The triad is located at the level of the A-I junction.

> Tc : Terminal cistern of sarcoplasmic reticulum.
> Tt : Transverse tubule.

Bottom: Cross section of a skeletal muscle fiber showing transversely sectioned A-, I- and Z-bands (A, I, Z). Mitochondria (m) are seen at the I-band level. Each myofibril is surrouded by sarcoplasmic reticulum (Sr) and the space between the myofibrils is mostly filled with numerous glycogen particles (Gl).

Top and Bottom: Material and method are the same as those of the picture on page 69. Top: ×52,000. Bottom: ×37,000.

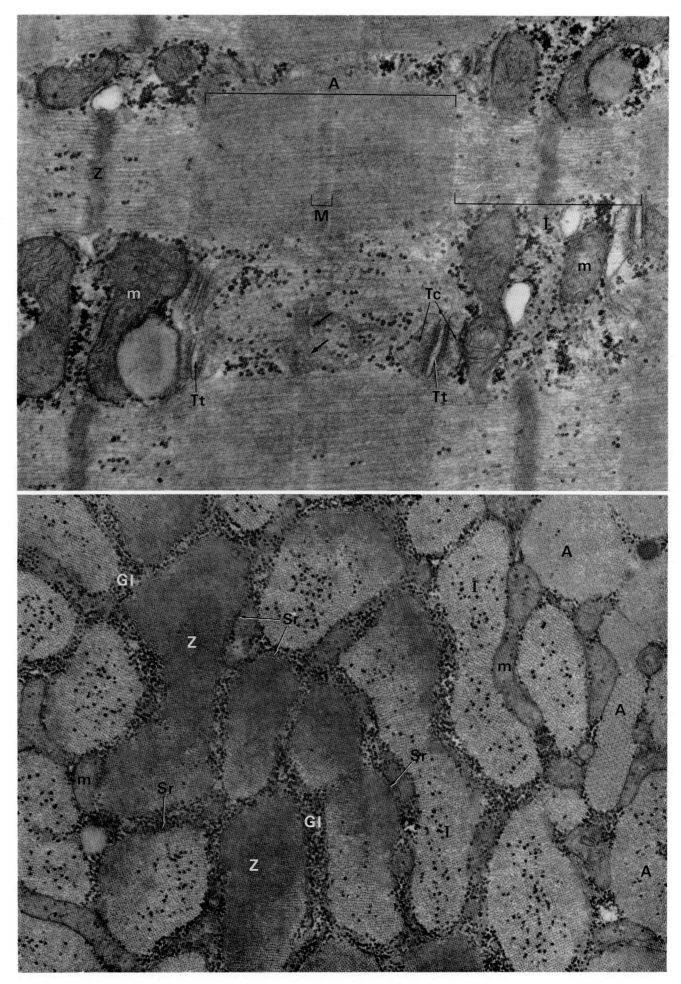

71

Muscle spindle

The muscle spindle is a proprioceptor which perceives the tension of the muscle to regulate reflectorily the movements of the muscle. It consists of a bundle of three to ten muscle fibers, or spindle fibers, which are smaller than the ordinary muscle fibers. They are enclosed by a thick sheath of connective tissue and supplied by afferent as well as efferent nerve fibers.

Top: A transverse section of a muscle spindle at the polar segment, the slender polar portion of the muscle spindle. Besides four spindle fibers (Sf), a few blood vessels (Bv) and myelinated nerve fibers (Nf) are enclosed within the connective tissue capsule which consists of concentrically-arranged thin cytoplasm sheets of fibrocytes (Fc) and collagenous fibers.

    Art: Arteriole.
    N: Nucleus of the spindle fiber.

Bottom: Cross section of a spindle fiber at the polar segment showing motor endings (Ne) in the muscle spindle. The ending is encapsulated in the cell of Schwann (Sch).

    A, I, Z: Cross section of myofibrils at levels of A-, I- and Z-bands.
    Fc: Fibrocyte surrounding the spindle fiber and nerve endings.

Top and Bottom: Material and method are the same as those of the picture on page 69. Top: ×2,100. Bottom: ×8,000.

REFERENCE:

RUMPELT, H.J. und H. SCHMALBRUCH: Zur Morphologie der Bauelemente von Muskelspindeln bei Mensch und Ratte. Z. Zellforsch., *102*: 601–630, 1969.

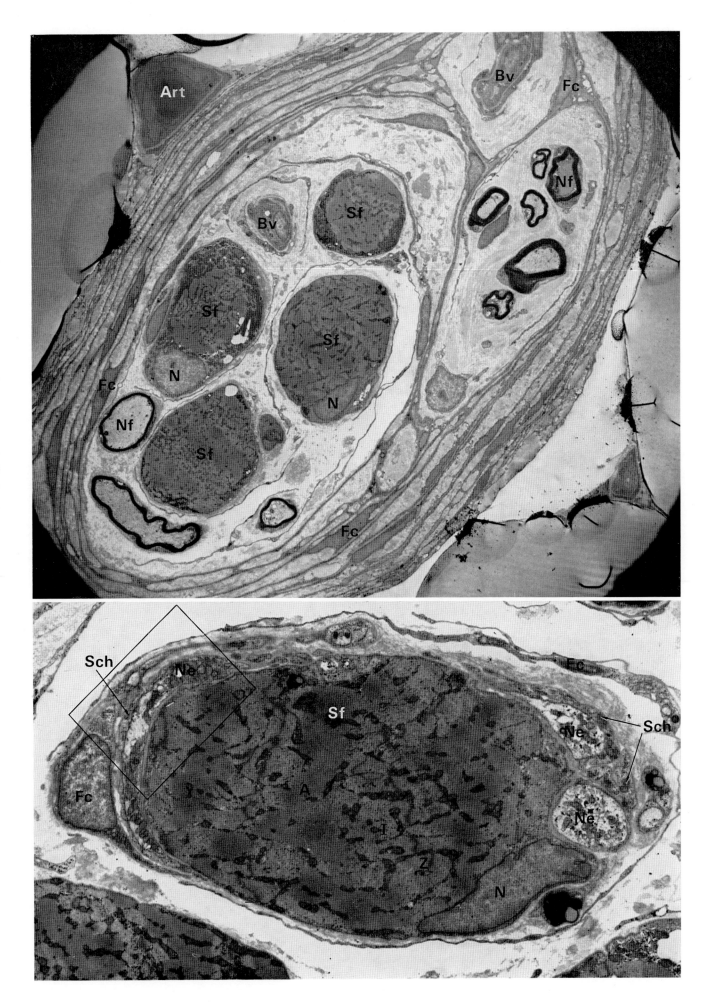

Motor nerve ending in the muscle spindle (Top)

This is a closer view of the small area enclosed in the rectangle in the bottom picture on page 73. The nerve ending containing a number of synaptic vesicles (Sy) and mitochondria (m) is separated from the muscle fiber by a wide gap which is filled with a substance of medium electron density (*). A Schwann cell (Sch) surrounds the nerve terminal on the opposite side of the muscle fiber.

A, I, Z : Cut ends of the myofibrils at different levels.
Fc : Fibrocyte.

Satellite cell (Bottom)

The satellite cell (Sc) is a flattened cell occupying a shallow dent in the surface of the skeletal muscle fiber. It is thought to be a remaining and resting fibroblast and becomes proliferative in the regeneration of the skeletal muscle fiber. The satellite cell applies to the surface of the muscle fiber on one side and, on the opposite side, is covered by a surface coat in common with the muscle fiber. The scanty cytoplasm of the satellite cell contains few cell organelles.

Gl : Glycogen particle.
m : Mitochondrion.

Top and Bottom: Material and method are the same as those of the picture on page 69. Top: ×30,000. Bottom: ×26,000.

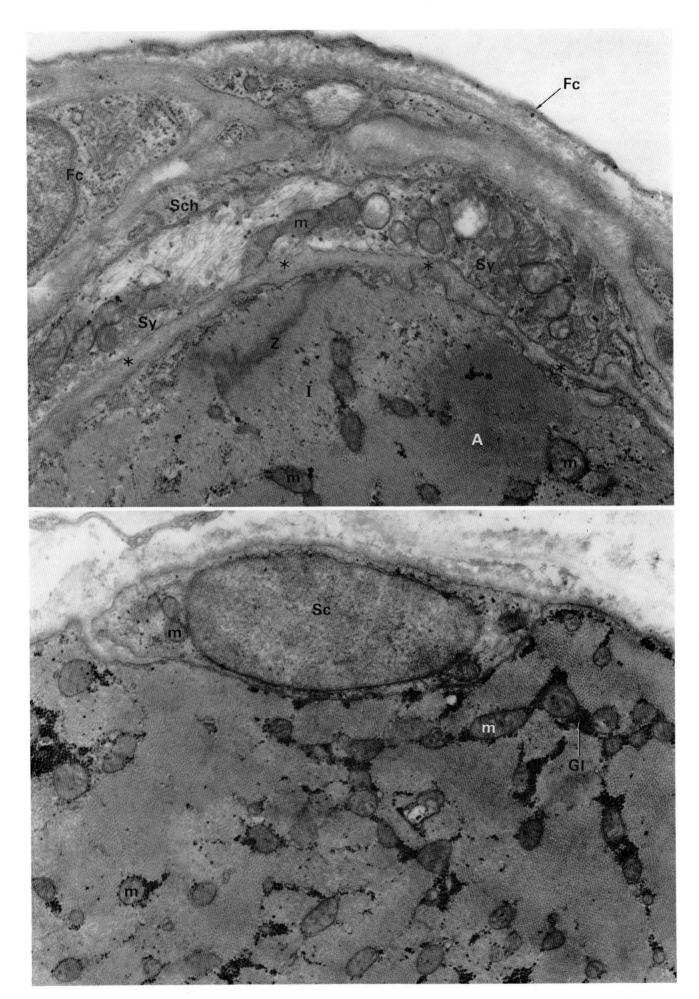

MUSCULAR TISSUE

Cardiac muscle

The cardiac muscle occurs in the myocardium of the heart and the walls of the large veins joining the heart. The cardiac muscle cells, the unit structure of the cardiac muscle, contract rhythmically and automatically even in a separated and cultured state. Each cardiac muscle cell has one or two nuclei which, like those of the smooth muscle fiber, are located in the center of the cell. Myofibrils of the cardiac muscle cell show a pattern of striation with A-, I-, M- and Z-bands identical to that of the skeletal muscle fiber. The cardiac muscle cell is richer in sarcoplasm and mitochondria than the skeletal muscle fiber.

The cardiac muscle fiber consisting of several cardiac muscle cells tends to branch and anastomose with adjacent cardiac muscle fibers to form a complex three-dimentional reticulum. The intercalated discs which are seen as peculiar transverse dark-lines in light microscopy are the site of the junction of the cardiac muscle cells. Connective tissue containing abundant blood capillaries occupies the space between the meshwork of cardiac muscle fibers.

Top: Longitudinal section of cardiac muscle cells. The orientation of the nucleus (N) with the prominent nucleoli is elongated longitudinally. The sarcoplasm contains myofibrils among which mitochondria (m) and glycogen particles are dispersed. In the paranuclear region, relatively well-developed Golgi complexes (Go) are seen and an intercalated disc (*) is seen at the top of this picture.

Bottom: Cross section of cardiac muscle cells. The nucleus with a distinct nucleolus (Nu) is located in the center of the muscle cell. In the sarcoplasm, large mitochondria (m) and lipid droplets (Ld) are seen dispersed among myofibrils cut at different levels. In the lower left corner, where the muscle cells are applied together, desmosomes (d) and tight junctions (arrows) are discernible.

A, I, Z: A-, I- and Z-bands of the sarcomere.
Cap: Blood capillary.
Fc: Fibrocyte in the connective tissue.
Ly: Lysosome.

Top and Bottom: Left auricle of the heart of a 12-year-old male with tetralogy of Fallot. Specimen obtained during open-heart surgery to prepare for the insertion of the polyethylene tube in order to connect the artificial heart-lung machine. Cacodylate-buffered 2.5% glutaraldehyde fixation followed by 1.0% osmium tetroxide post-fixation. Uranyl acetate and lead tartarate staining. Top: ×6,500. Bottom: ×8,500.

REFERENCES:

Batting, C. G. and F. N. Low: The ultrastructure of human cardiac muscle and its associated tissue space. Amer. J. Anat., *108*: 199–229, 1961.

Lannigan, R. A. and S. A. Zaki: Ultrastructure of the myocardium of the atrial appendage. Brit. Heart J., *28*: 796–807, 1966.

Smith, J. R., T. H. Burford and A. D. Chiquoine: Electron microscopic observations of the ventricular heart muscle of man obtained by surgical biopsy during thoracotomy. Exp. Cell Res., *20*: 228–232, 1960.

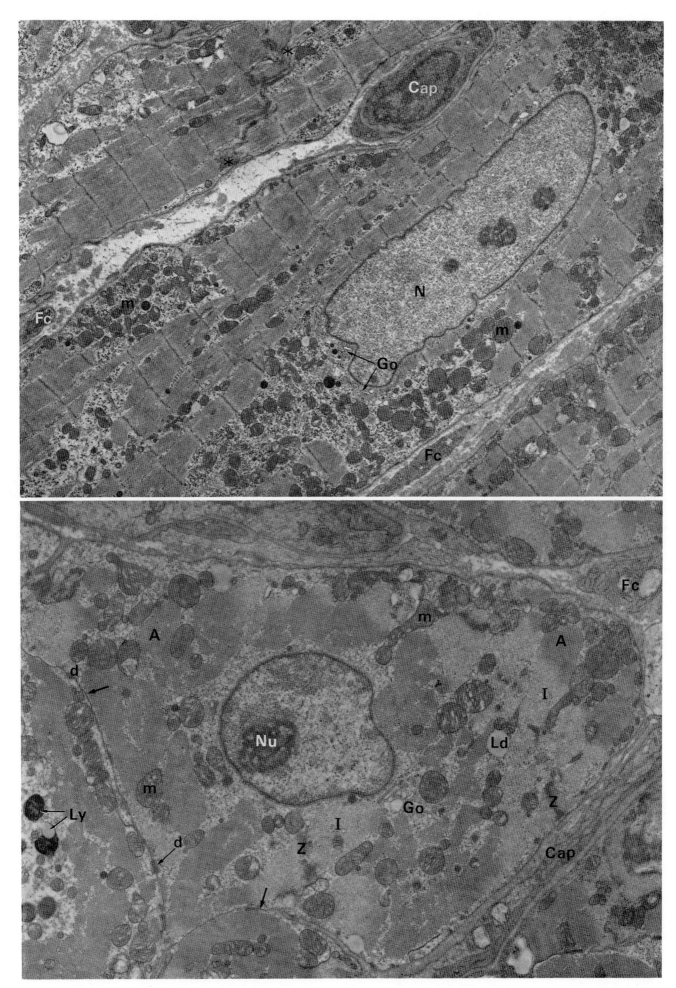

MUSCULAR TISSUE

Longitudinal section of a cardiac muscle fiber

Within a muscle fiber, myofibrils with characteristic cross striation of A-, I- and Z-bands are gathered into bundles. The darkest lines, the Z-bands, are the boundaries of the functional and structural segments of the muscle fiber, the sarcomeres (Sa). Mitochondria (m), glycogen particles (Gl) and a few profiles of sarcoplasmic reticulum occupy the cleft between myofibrils. The transverse tubules, which are seen at the A-I junction level in the skeletal muscle fiber, are at the Z-band level in the cardiac muscle cell (arrows). The cell membrane (sarcolemma) covered by a thick coating is attached to elastic fibres at the places marked by asterisks.

Material and method are the same as those of the picture on page 77. ×21,000.

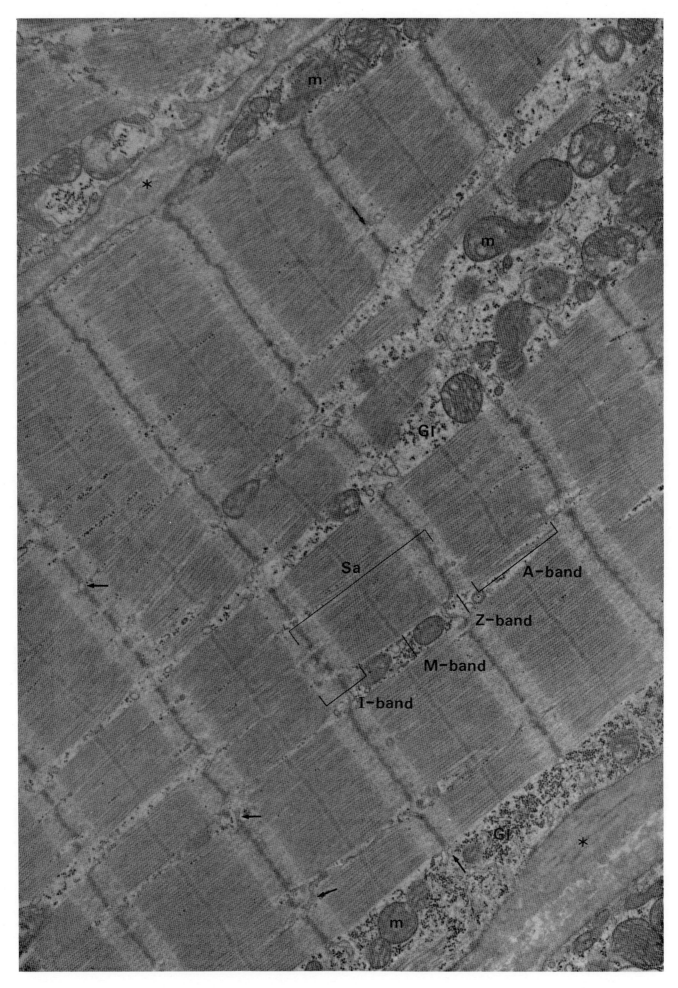

79

Sarcomere of the cardiac muscle fiber

Top: This is a longitudinal section of a cardiac muscle fiber showing the arrangement of thick (myosin) and thin (actin) filaments in the sarcomere. The I-band consists of only thin filaments and its middle is occupied by the Z-band. The A-band is the zone where thick filaments are seen. At either end, the A-band contains both thick and thin filaments. The middle of the A-band is called M-band.

Tt: Transverse tubules located at the Z-band level.

Bottom: Cross section of a cardiac muscle fiber showing the regular, ordered arrangements of thick and thin filaments in the myofibrils at different levels.

N: Nucleus.
Nm: Nuclear membrane.
Sr: Sarcoplasmic reticulum.
Z: Z-band.

Top and Bottom: Material and method are the same as those of the picture on page 77. Top: ×51,000. Bottom: ×67,000.

REFERENCES:

CHIBA, T. and A. YAMAUCHI: On the fine structure of the nerve terminals in the human myocardium. Z. Zellforsch., *108*: 324–338, 1970.

NELSON, D. A. and E. S. BENSON: On the structural continuities of the transverse tubular system of rabbit and human myocardial cells. J. Cell Biol., *16*: 297–313, 1963.

STEIN, A. A., F. THIBODEAU and A. STRANAHAN: Electron microscope studies of human myocardium. J. Amer. med. Ass., *128*: 537–540, 1962.

YAMAUCHI, A.: Electron microscopic observations on the development of S–A and A–V nodal tissues in the human embryonic heart. Z. Anat. Entw.-gesch., *124*: 562–587, 1965.

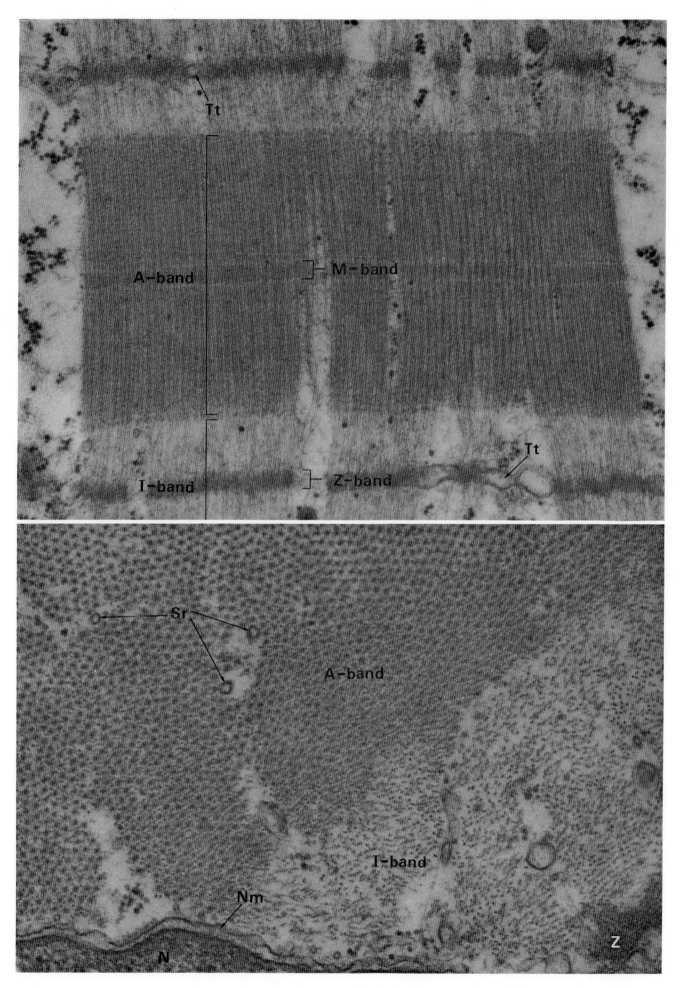

81

Intercalated disc of the cardiac muscle

At the level of light microscopy, one of the most disputable problems was whether the heart was a syncytium or a mass of cells. Though the cardiac muscle was known to be segmented by transverse markings called intercalated discs which were blackened by silver nitrate and stained by some dyes such as iron haematoxylin, it was not known whether they corresponded to cell boundaries or not. Electron microscopy revealed that the heart consists of a great number of independent cardiac muscle cells and that the intercalated discs are nothing but the site of end-to-end attachments of the cells. The intercalated disc consists of numerous tight junctions and desmosomes. The former are believed to be the device for the conduction of excitation from cell to cell, while the latter are the specialization for the cohesion of the cardiac muscle cells.

Top: Longitudinal section of parts of two cardiac muscle cells showing the junction between them. The typical zigzag pattern of the intercalated disc is seen.

Bottom: Cross section of several cardiac muscle cells showing intercalated discs consisting of desmosomes (d) and tight junctions (Tj). Myofibrils cut in cross section at various levels are also seen. From this picture, it is obvious that thin actin filaments terminate in desmosomes.

A, I, Z : A-, I- and Z-bands of the sarcomere.
Gl : Glycogen particle.
m : Mitochondrion.
Sr : Sarcoplasmic reticulum.

Top and Bottom: Material and method are the same as those of the picture on page 77. Top: ×36,000. Bottom: ×38,000.

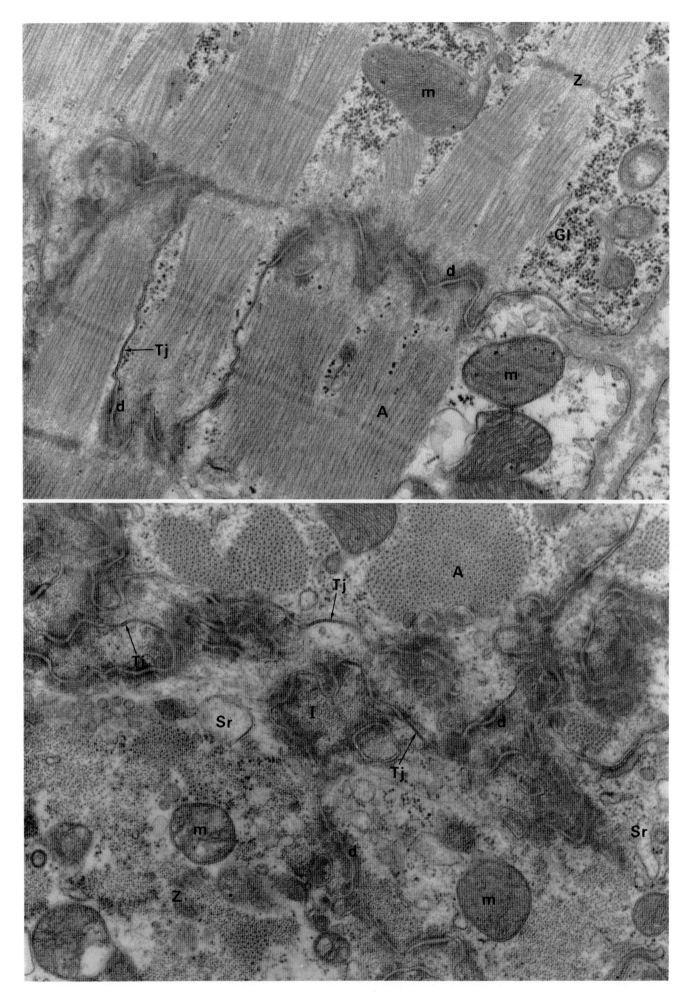

NERVOUS TISSUE

Autonomic ganglion

The autonomic ganglion consists of groups of nerve cells and bundles of nerve fibers associated with scarce connective tissue containing blood vessels.

The autonomic nerve cell is usually multipolar in shape. In this micrograph which was obtained from a lumbar sympathetic ganglion of a 7-month fetus, the perikaryon or cell body of a nerve cell projects four cytoplasmic processes (Cp). The nerve cell contains a large, round nucleus with a centrically-located prominent nucleolus (Nu). Chromatin is so scanty that the nucleus as a whole looks like a clear vesicle. The cytoplasm contains stacks of granular endoplasmic reticulum which form characteristic Nissl bodies (Ni), numerous profiles of Golgi complexes (Go), mitochondria (m) and a number of lysosomes (Ly).

The perikaryon of the nerve cell is completely surrounded by a capsule of satellite cells (Sat) which are apparently identical in fine structure with Schwann cells (Sch). The nuclei of both satellite cells and Schwann cells are small, elongated and dense, and have small nucleoli. The scarce cytoplasm of these cells contains centrioles (c), mitochondria, Golgi complexes and other usual cell organelles concentrated around the nuclei.

Numerous collagenous fibrils and fibroblasts (Fb) are dispersed between the nerve cell and nerve fibers.

Cap: Blood capillary.
Nf: Non-myelinated nerve fiber.
Pc: Pericyte of the blood capillary.

From a lumbar sympathetic ganglion of a 7-month fetus (♂, 1,850 g). Fixation in phosphate-buffered 2.5% glutaraldehyde followed by post-fixation in 1.0% osmium tetroxide solution. Uranyl acetate and lead tartarate staining. ×4,000.

REFERENCES:

CRAVIOTO, H.: The role of Schwann cells in the development of human peripheral nerves. An electron microscopic study. J. Ultrastr. Res., *12*: 634–651, 1965.

GAMBLE, H. J.: Further electron microscope studies of human foetal peripheral nerves. J. Anat., *100*: 487–502, 1966.

GAMBLE, H. J. and R. A. EAMES: An electron microscope study of the connective tissues of human peripheral nerve. J. Anat., *98*: 655–663, 1964.

GAMBLE, H. J. and R. A. EAMES: Electron microscopy of human spinal-nerve roots. Arch. Neurol., *14*: 50–53, 1966.

OHSUGA, N., S. SHIONOYA, K. KAMIYA and M. HOSHINO: An electron microscopic study of the human sympathetic ganglion cell. I. Inclusion bodies. J. Electron Microsc., *15*: 26–27, 1966.

PICK, J., C. de LEMOS and C. GERDIN: The fine structure of sympathetic neurons in man. J. comp. Neurol., *122*: 19–67, 1964.

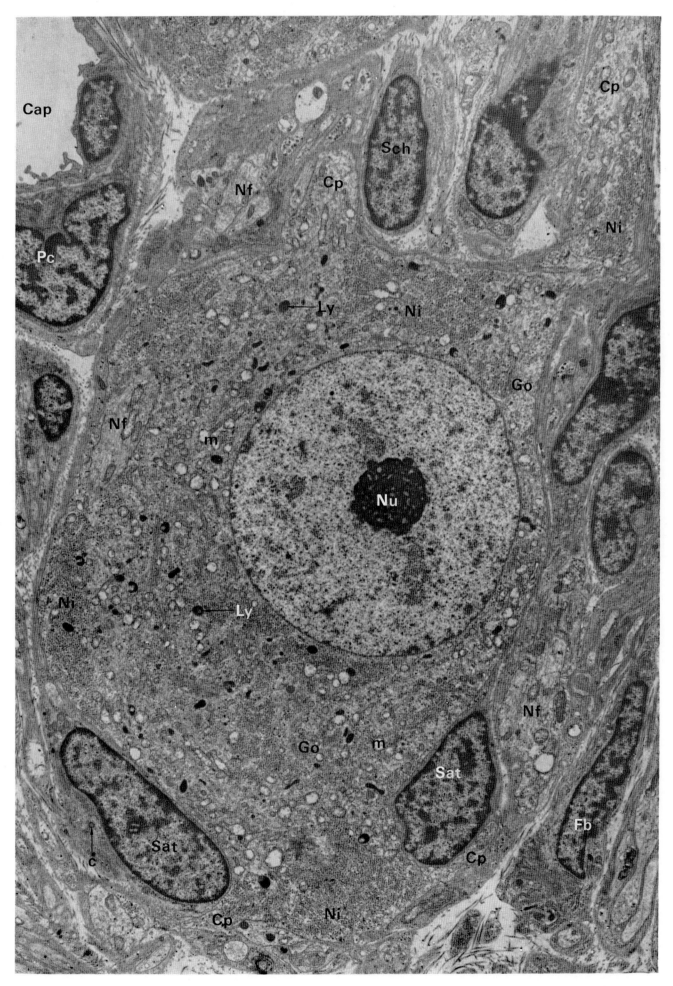

85

Perikaryon of a pyramidal neuron in the cerebral cortex

The nucleus of the nerve cell, like that of other cells, is bounded by a double-layered envelope which is provided with numerous nuclear pores (arrows). A large, rounded nucleolus (Nu) is seen. In the cytoplasm are small Nissl bodies (Ni) consisting of stacks of granular endoplasmic reticulum, many clusters of free ribosomes, Golgi complexes (Go), mitochondria (m), lysosomes (Ly) and microtubules (t). At the right side of this picture is the neuropil containing several profiles of axo-dendritic synapses (Sy) and processes of neurons and glial cells.

From the polymorphous layer of the right temporal lobe of a 63-year-old man with right hemisphere glioma. Obtained during surgical operation for the insertion of polyethylene tube through which the fluid of the tumor was inhaled. Phosphate-buffered 2.5% glutaraldehyde fixation followed by 1.0% osmium tetroxide post-fixation. Stained with uranyl acetate and lead tartarate solution. ×14,000.

REFERENCE:

GONATAS, N. K.: The significance of " pale " neurons in human cortical biopsies. An electron microscopic study. J. neurol. Pathol. exp. Neurol., *25*: 637–645, 1966.

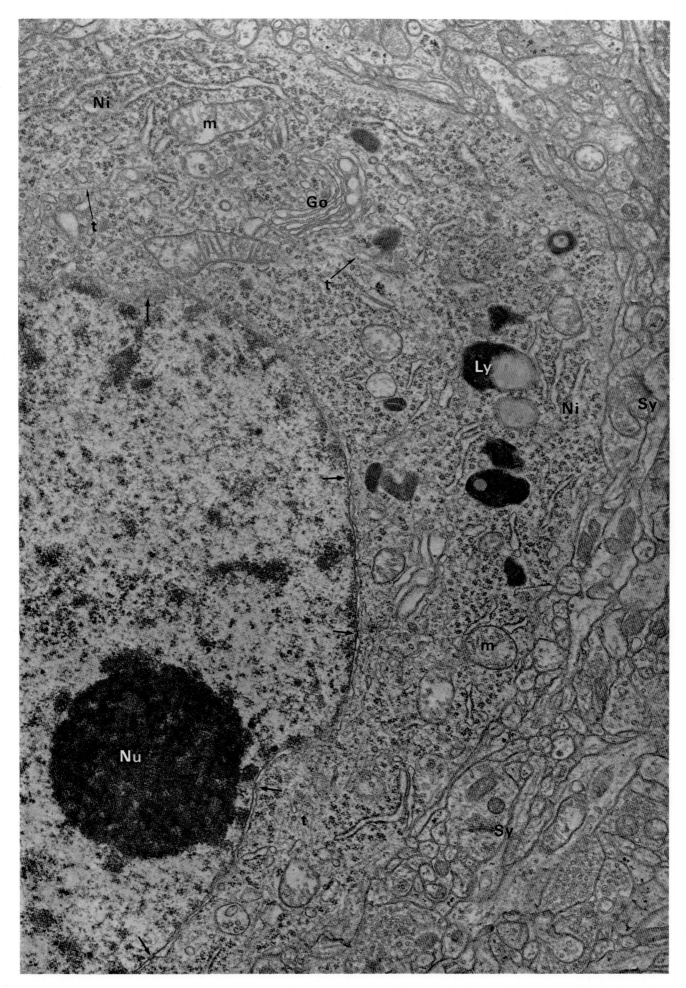

87

Nissl substance of the sympathetic ganglion cell (Top)

In light microscopic preparations, the cytoplasm of nerve cells contains intensely basophilic bodies. The Nissl bodies, as they are called, have been one of the criteria of nerve cells, though their distribution, size and shape differ from cell to cell. Electron microscopic studies have revealed that Nissl bodies are no more than stacks of granular endoplasmic reticulum plus numerous free ribosomes. It is evidenced that the RNA contained in the granular endoplasmic reticulum and free ribosomes is intensely basophilic and is stained by basic dyes such as thionin and toluidine blue.

This picture is, for the most part, occupied by Nissl substance consisting of cisterns of granular endoplasmic reticulum and clusters of free ribosomes. In the lower left corner part of a Golgi complex (Go) is seen. Microtubules are scattered between cell organelles (arrows).

From a lumbar sympathetic ganglion of a 6-month fetus (♀, 600 g). Method for specimen preparation is the same as that of the picture on page 85. ×58,000.

Oligodendroglia and cerebral capillary (Bottom)

This picture shows a portion of the cerebral cortex containing a capillary (Cap) and two oligodendroglia (Ol). One of the latter has dark cytoplasm and the other posesses rather light cytoplasm. The nucleus of an oligodendroglia usually shows clumpings of chromatin at the periphery. Unlike the astroglia, the oligodendroglia contains only a small number of cytoplasmic filaments. Note a long process which extends from the cell body of the dark oligodendroglia. The capillary in the cerebral cortex has a continuous endothelium and a surrounding continuous basal lamina (Bl). Around the capillary, processes of astroglia are seen (∗).

Ly: Lysosome in the process of oligodendroglia.
My: Myelinated nerve fiber.
Nu: Nucleolus.

Material and method are the same as those of the picture on page 87. ×7,500.

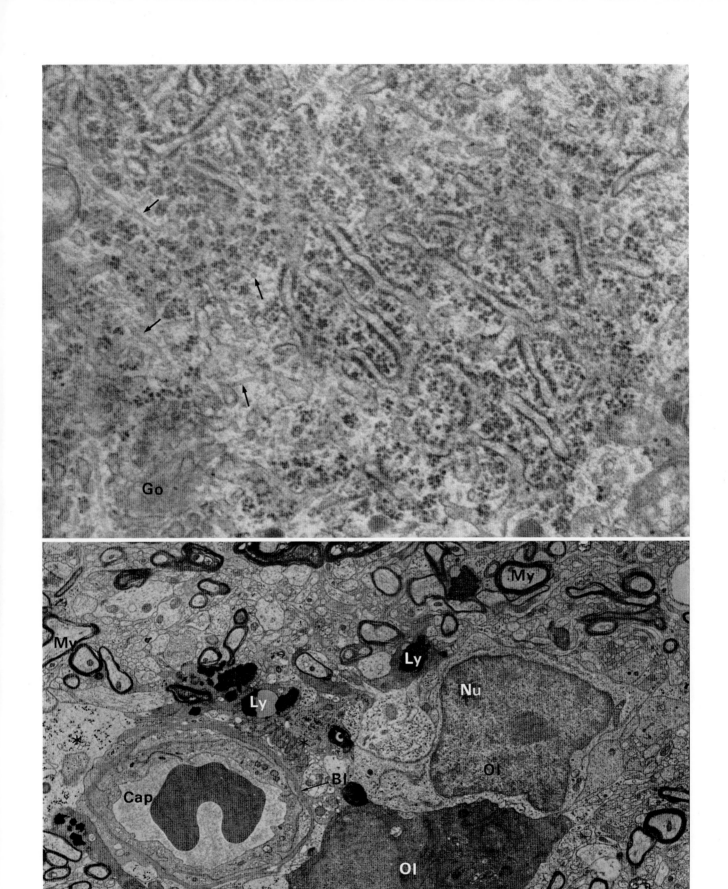

89

Astroglia (Top)

The outline of an astroglia is very irregular and seems to follow the contours of the elements in the surrounding neuropil. The nucleus appears homogeneous in density. The cytoplasm contains relatively sparse cell organelles: several mitochondria (m), Golgi complexes (Go), irregularly-shaped lysosomes (Ly) and a few strands of granular endoplasmic reticulum are present. Abundant cytoplasmic filaments occupy the majority of the cytoplasm.

f: Cytoplasmic filaments.
My: Myelinated nerve fiber.
Nu: Nucleolus.
Ol: Oligodendroglia.

Axo-dendritic synapses and a fibrous astroglia (Bottom)

The upper portion of this picture is occupied by an astroglia containing a large lysosome (Ly), profiles of Golgi complexes (Go), mitochondria (m), a few strands of granular endoplasmic reticulum (Er) and abundant cytoplasmic filaments (f).

Crossing the lower field is a longitudinally-sectioned dendrite (Dr) which has a cluster of microtubules or neurotubules in the cytoplasm. An axon terminal (At_1) containing numerous synaptic vesicles makes a synaptic contact with this dendrite. One of the other axon terminals (At_2) synapses with a profile of the dendrite on the left side.

As: Process of an astroglia.
At: Axon terminal.
Ol: Oligodendroglia.

Top and Bottom: Material and method are the same as those of the picture on page 87. Top: ×7,500. Bottom: ×18,000.

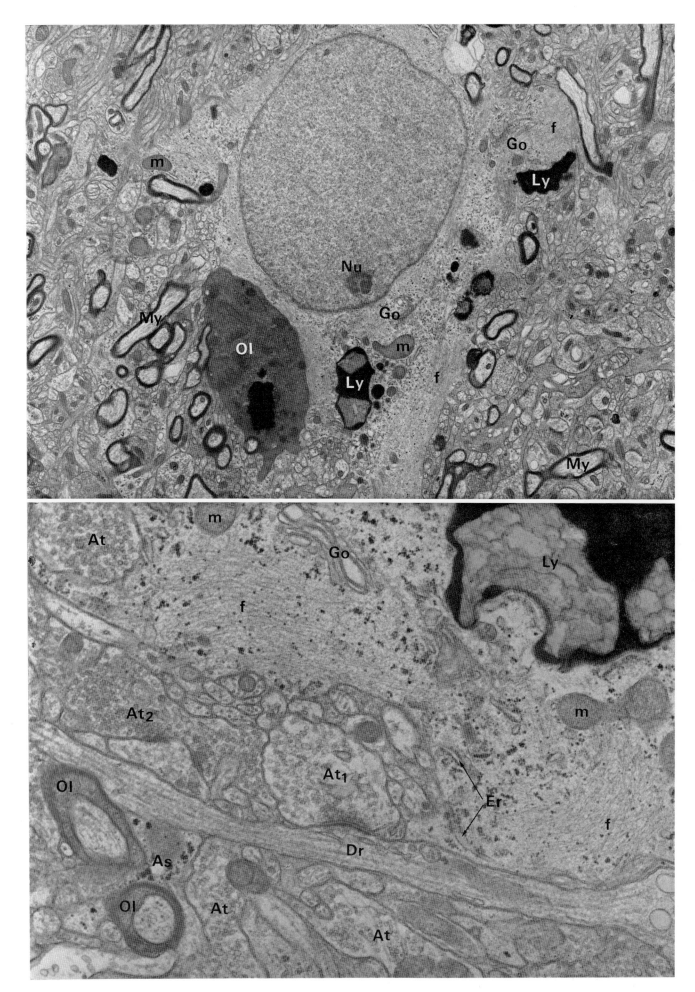

91

Neuropil in the cerebral cortex

In this micrograph three profiles of axo-dendritic synapses are seen ($Sy_{1, 2, 3}$). The axon terminals ($At_{1, 2, 3}$) contain numerous synaptic vesicles. At the synaptic area the cell membranes of the axon terminal and dendrite come into apposition with a narrow space, and dense filamentous substance in the adjacent cytoplasm is gathered toward it. In the dendrite shown in the center of this picture a spine apparatus (Sp) consisting of cisterns of smooth membrane is seen. Note abundant microtubules in this dendrite. The astrocytic process (As) is characterized by the presence of glycogen-like dense particles. The arrow indicates a Schmidt-Lanterman's incision in the myelin sheath.

m: Mitochondrion.

Material and method are the same as those of the picture on page 87. ×41,000.

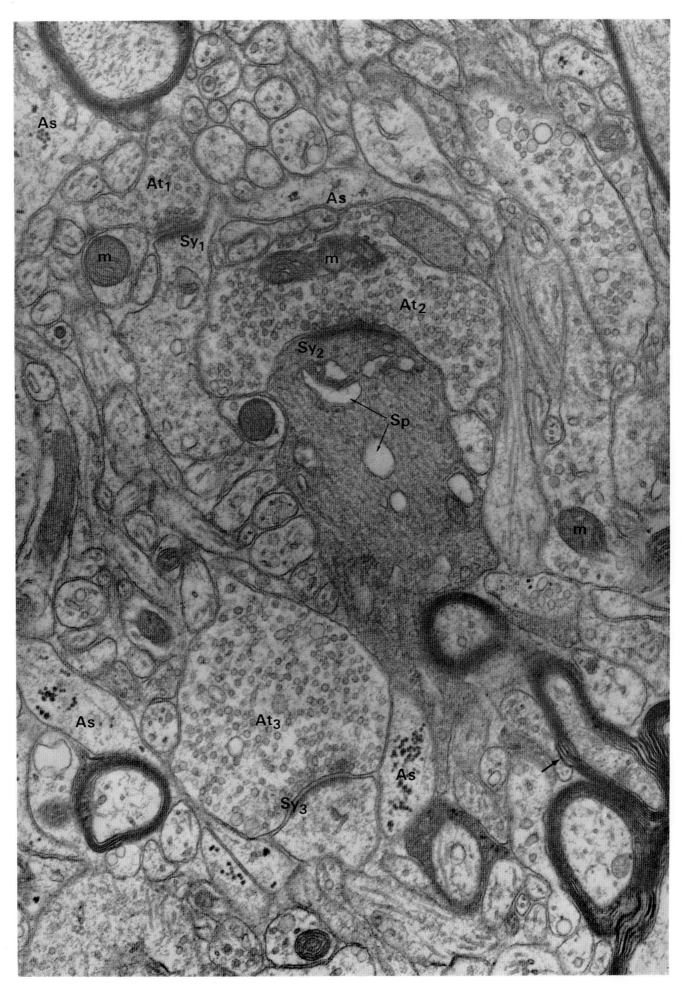

93

The tooth germ consists of two components: enamel organ and dental papilla. The enamel organ develops from a mass of ectodermal cells derived from the primitive oral epithelium. It consists of four layers: outer enamel epithelium, stellate reticulum, stratum intermedium and ameloblastic layer. The ameloblasts are extremely elongated cells destined to form the enamel of the tooth. The dental papilla is of mesenchymal origin. The dental pulp is formed from this tissue, and covering the surface of the pulp are large epitheloid cells, odontoblasts, which become differentiated and produce dentin.

Stellate reticulum (Top)

The stellate reticulum occupies the middle part of the enamel organ and consists of stellate cells and wide intercellular space. Desmosomes (d) and tight junctions connect the tapered cytoplasmic processes of adjacent cells giving them a stellate appearance. The cells further possess many microvillous processes (p). The cytoplasm of these cells contains numerous mitochondria (m), lysosomal granules (Ly), bundles of tonofilaments (f), scattered profiles of granular endoplasmic reticulum (Er), numerous free ribosomes, Golgi complexes (Go), lipid droplets and glycogen particles (Gl). The large intercellular space (Is) is filled with a gelatinous substance rich in mucopolysaccharides.

N: Nucleus.

Stratum intermedium (Bottom)

The stratum intermedium is the layer of enamel organ immediately outside of the ameloblastic layer.

The cells of this layer and those of the stellate reticulum have a similar ultrastructure in terms of cytoplasmic organelles. The cells of this stratum contact the basal ends of ameloblasts (Am) by desmosomes (d) and tight junctions (Tj) and they are more closely packed than the cells of the stellate reticulum.

Top and Bottom: From a tooth germ of a 7-month fetus (♂, 1,850 g). Fixation with 2.5% glutaraldehyde in phosphate buffer followed by 1.0% osmium tetroxide post-fixation. Uranyl acetate and lead citrate staining. Top: ×15,000. Bottom: ×18,000. (Photographs courtesy of Dr. H. OZAWA)

REFERENCES:

STACK, M. V. and R. W. FEARNHEAD (ed.): Tooth enamel. John Wright & Sons, Bristol, 1965.

MILES, A. E. W. (ed.): Structure and chemical organization of teeth. I, II. Academic Press, New York, 1967.

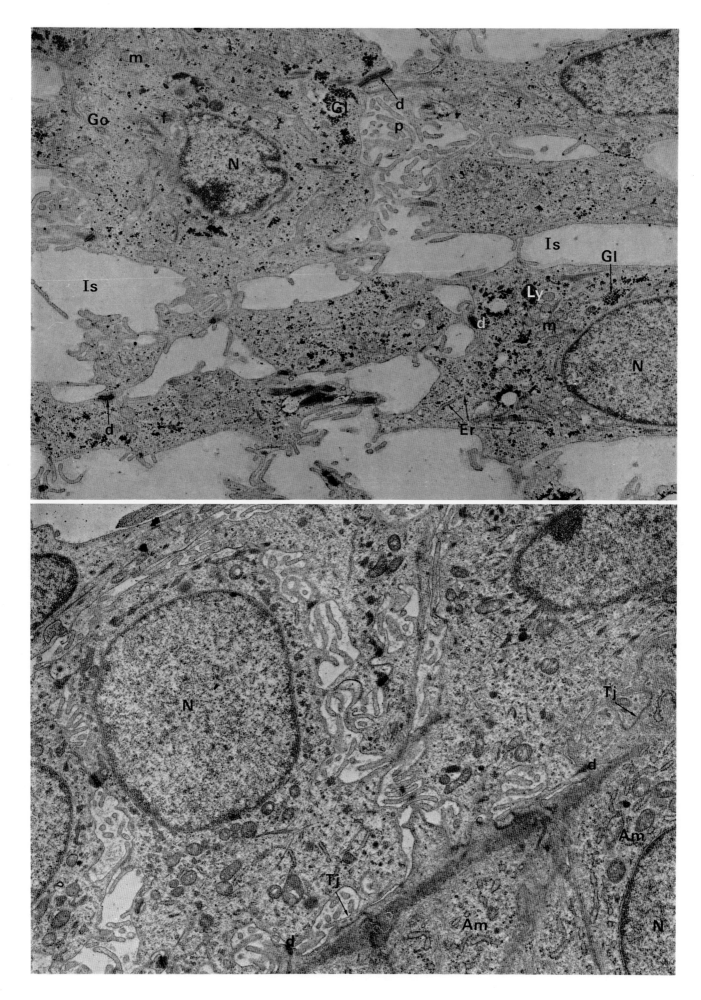

Ameloblast

Ameloblasts are the cells lining the innermost layer of the enamel organ. The active ameloblasts are high-columnar in shape and possess a characteristic Tomes' process at their distal end.

Top: A longitudinal section of ameloblasts actively engaged in enamel formation is shown. The nuclus (N) is strongly shifted toward the basal end of the cell. Golgi complexes (Go) are located in the center, and the granular endoplasmic reticulum (Er) occurs at all levels but most noticeably at the distal end of the cell. Mitochondria (m) are scattered throughout the cytoplasm. A Tomes' process (Tp) constitutes the distal extremity of an ameloblast. Protruding into the enamel (En), the Tomes' process give the enamel surface an uneven, serrated appearance. The ameloblasts are joined to their neighbours by desmosomes (d), tight junctions and proximal and distal terminal bars (pTb, dTb).

Tooth germ of a 7-month fetus (♂, 1,450 g). Fixation with 2.5% glutaraldehyde in phosphate buffer, decalcified with EDTA, then followed by 1.0% osmium tetroxide post-fixation. Uranyl acetate and lead citrate staining. ×4,500. (Photograph courtesy of Dr. H. OZAWA)

Bottom: This micrograph shows a Golgi area of a mature ameloblast. The Golgi complex (Go) is large and composed of stacks of cisterns and associated vesicles. Numerous secretion granules (Sg), coated vesicles (Cv) and a multivesicular body (Mvb) are present in the Golgi area. Microtubules (t) and tonofilaments (f) can be seen coursing in an axial direction within the cytoplasm. Arrows indicate that coated vesicles are budding from the endoplasmic reticulum (Er).

Material and method are the same as those of the top picture, except decalcification. ×27,000. (Photograph courtesy of Dr. H. OZAWA)

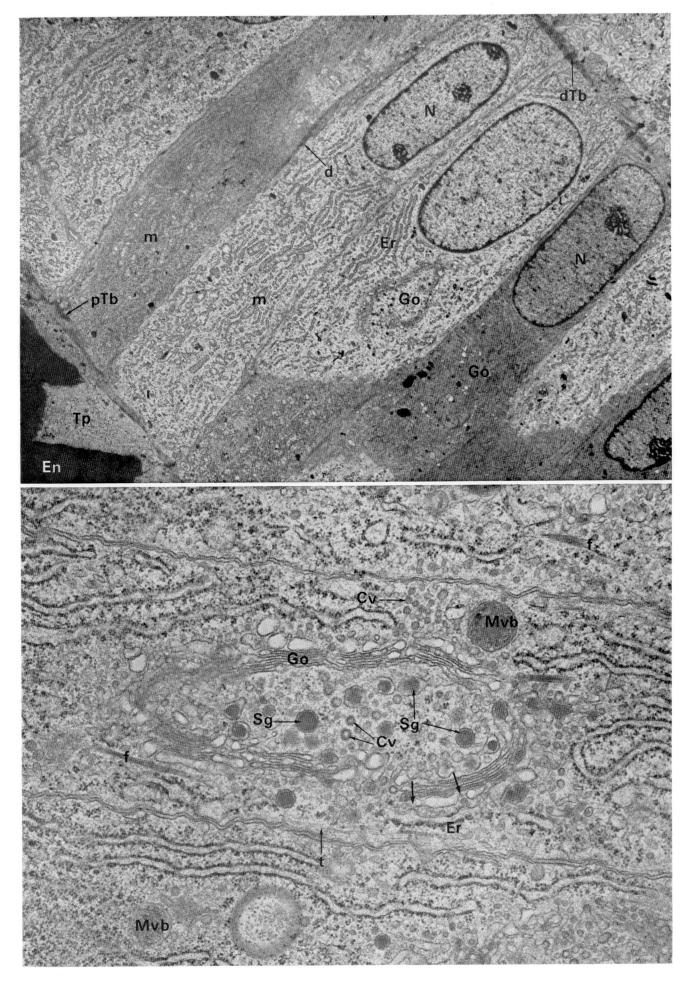

97

DEVELOPING TOOTH

Enamel rod and Tomes' process of the ameloblast

The enamel of the tooth is formed of a multitude of enamel rods or prisms which are tall columns of calcified material that extend from the dentino-enamel junction to the surface of the enamel.

Tomes' processes, the tapering projections of the ameloblasts are thought to play a very important role in the elaboration of the enamel matrix and in the reabsorption of a portion of the enamel matrix once deposited. It is accepted that one cell is responsible for the formation of one enamel prism.

Top left: Cross section of enamel rods. In this micrograph, the enamel rods appear as "keyhole or tadpole-tail" structures. The peripheral shell of each enamel rod is known to be less calcified and richer in organic matter than the rod substance. This area is referred to as the rod or prism sheath (Rs).

After decalcification with EDTA, the mineral components of enamel, such as apatite crystals, are completely eliminated; but in an immature enamel as in the case of this micrograph, a considerable amount of organic material remains and is seen as filamentous forms arranged in a fur-like pattern.

Top right: Tomes' process of an ameloblast and developing enamel rod. The Tomes' process of an ameloblast consists of a proximal part which extends the region of the terminal bars (Tb) to the mineralization front, and a distal part which projects into the surface of the enamel. The process contains coated vesicles, dense secretion granules (Sg), numerous smooth vesicles, microtubules, fine filaments and multivesicular bodies. Neither mitochondria nor granular endoplasmic reticulum can be found here. The secretion granules bounded by a slightly wrinkled membrane are believed to be derived from the Golgi complex of the ameloblast.

The enamel at this stage (En), demineralized with EDTA, shows a rich content of organic matter which appears as fibriles arranged between the vacancies left by the removed enamel crystals.

Top left and right: Material and method are the same as those of the top micrograph on page 97. Top left: ×19,000. Top right: ×10,000. (Photographs courtesy of Dr. H. Ozawa)

Bottom: This micrograph is from a section of an undecalcified tooth germ. The Tomes' process (Tp) contains numerous small vesicles, a few dense secreting granules (Sg) and fine filaments. So-called stippled material is located around the process and in the intercellular space of ameloblasts at the level of Tomes' processes (arrows).

Enamel rods (En) constituted of fibrillar enamel crystals which indicate the orientation of the movement of ameloblasts are continuous to the Tomes' process.

Tooth germ of a 7-month fetus (♂, 1,850 g). Phosphate-buffered 2.5% glutaraldehyde fixation followed by 1.0% osmium tetroxide post-fixation. Undecalcified. Uranyl acetate and lead citrate staining. ×28,000. (Photograph courtesy of Dr. H. Ozawa)

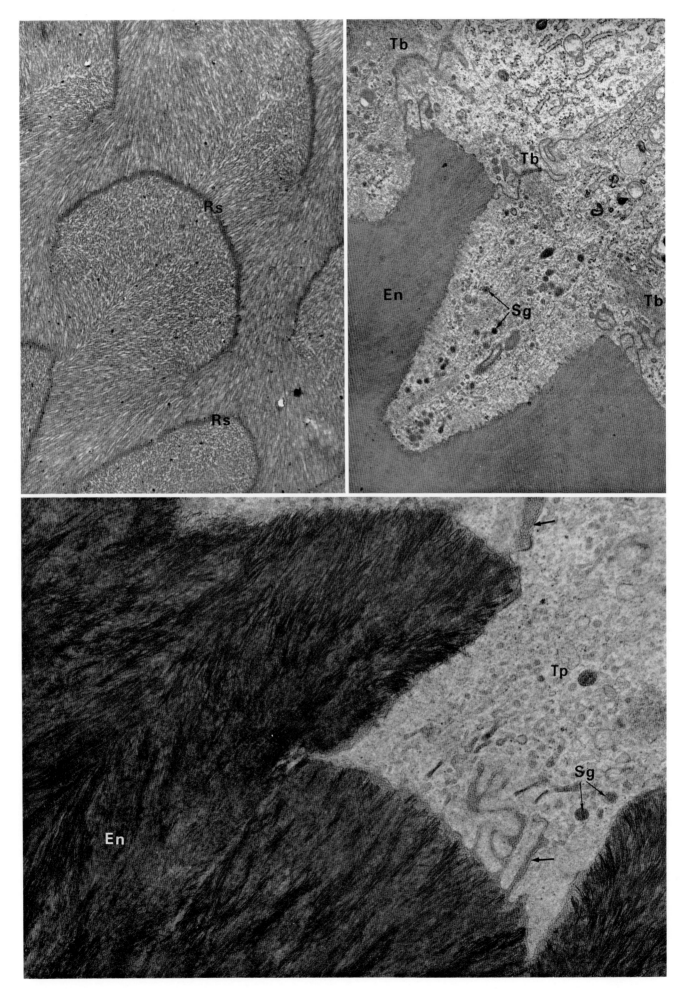

Dentin

Top : A section of undecalcified tooth germ shows developing dentin in an early stage of mineralization. Acid-resistant crystals after uranyl acetate staining can be seen in the intertubular matrix, whereas they are more densely packed in the peritubular region (Pt) which becomes highly mineralized at a very early stage. An odontoblastic process (Op_1) in the mineralized dentin contains microtubules and fine filaments, whereas another process (Op_2) seen in the predential matrix still contains numerous dense vesicles.

The stipple-line indicates the boundary between the dentin and the predentin.

Pd : Predentin.
De : Dentin.

Undecalcified section of developing tooth germ of a 7-month fetus (♂, 1,450 g). Fixation with 2.5% glutaraldehyde in phosphate buffer followed by 1.0% osmium tetroxide solution. Uranyl acetate and lead citrate staining. ×19,000. (Photograph courtesy of Dr. H. Ozawa)

Bottom right : This micrograph of dentinal matrix in the region of the mineralization front shows irregularly-arranged collagenous fibers and the initiation of crystallization on some of them. Compare the forms of the crystals associated with the collagenous fibrils with those of the enamel crystals shown in the pictures on page 99.

Im : Intertubular matrix.

Undecalcified section of the same material as the top picture. Stained with lead citrate alone. ×42,000. (Photograph courtesy of Dr. H. Ozawa)

Bottom left : Decalcified dentin of a permanent tooth. A section of normal, decalcified dentin shows closely-packed, irregularly-arranged collagenous fibrils in the intertubular matrix, and a cross-sectioned dentinal tubule appears almost empty due to a poor fixation.

Upper first incisor of a 20-year-old male. Formalin fixation and EDTA decalcification. Unstained. ×15,000. (Photograph courtesy of Dr. H. Ozawa)

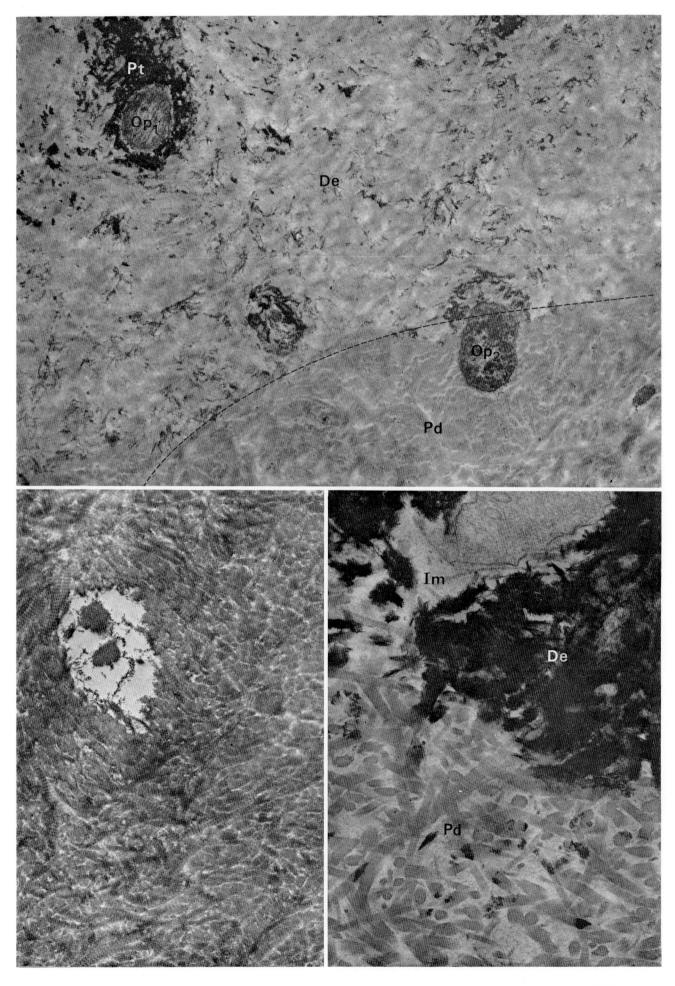

101

Odontoblast

Odontoblasts are large, columnar connective tissue cells lining the pulp cavity of a tooth. They are arranged in an epitheloid layer and have one or more slender cytoplasmic processes which project into the dentinal tubule. They play a leading part in the formation of the matrix of predentin, which consists mostly of collagenous fibrils, and also are important in the process of the calcification of the dentin.

The nucleus (N) of the odontoblast is elongated in shape and usually situated in the basal end of the cell. Scarce chromatin is gathered at the periphery, and the nucleolus is large and prominent. The cell body of the odontoblasts is filled with the cisterns of the endoplasmic reticulum (Er) distended with a moderately dense content except where a well-developed Golgi complex (Go) is situated above the nucleus. At least two types of cytoplasmic bodies can be seen around the Golgi complexes and in the odontoblastic process. One of them shows a lysosomal appearance (Ly), and another is represented by rod-shaped, polygonal bodies (Pb) containing a fibrous substance and dense granules. Numerous coated vesicles can also be seen in the Golgi region.

Microtubules and cytoplasmic filaments are observed coursing in an axial direction within the cytoplasm. Odontoblasts are joined to their neighbors by tight and desmosome-like junctions (Tj). Microvillous projections (Mv) are at the distal end of the cell and also occur between the cells to form intercellular canaliculi. Von Korff's fibers (Ko) consisting of bundles of fine filamentous material run between the odontoblasts and into the predentin.

Is: Intercellular space.

Lower deciduous molar tooth germ of a 7-month fetus (♂, 1,450 g). Fixation with 2.5% glutaraldehyde in phosphate buffer followed by 1.0% osmium tetroxide post-fixation. Uranyl acetate and lead citrate staining. ×18,000. (Photograph courtesy of Dr. H. Ozawa)

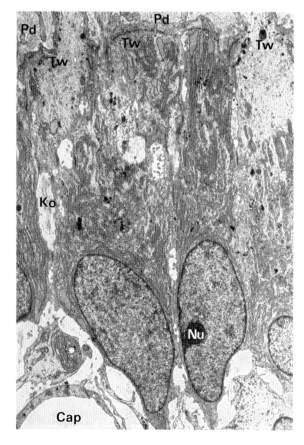

General aspects of mature odontoblasts.

Cap: Blood capillary.
Ko: Von Korff's fiber.
Nu: Nucleolus.
Tw: Terminal web.
Pd: Predentin.

Material and method are the same as those of the picture on page 103. ×3,000.

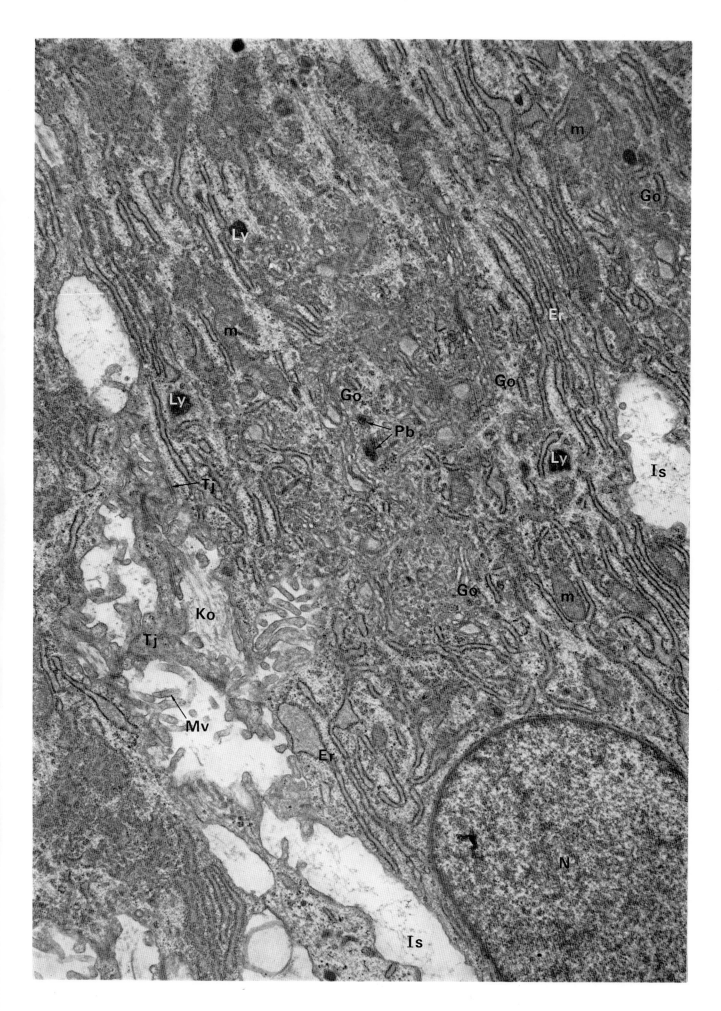

Odontoblastic process (Tomes' dentinal process)

The odontoblastic process is a cytoplasmic extension of the odontoblasts occupying a space in the dentin matrix known as the dentinal tubule.

The process lies beyond the terminal web layer of the odontoblast and contains several dense bodies (Db), a few multivesicular bodies (Mvb), smooth vesicles (v), coated vesicles (arrows), a tubular agranular endoplasmic reticulum (Ser), microtubules (t), fine filaments (f), and free ribosomes, but no granular endoplasmic reticulum, mitochondria or Golgi complex.

The extracellular space surrounding the base of the odontoblastic process is occupied by the predentinal matrix (Pd) which consists of collagenous fibrils in a reticular ground substance.

Von Korff's fibers (Ko) can be seen coursing in an axial direction along the odontoblastic process, and they pass through intercellular canaliculi that are formed by a separation of adjacent cell membranes which are not part of the junctional complex.

Top: Beginning of an odontoblastic process.

Bottom: Higher magnified micrograph of the odontoblastic process. Note the branching of the odontoblastic process (*).

Top and Bottom: Material and method are the same as those of the picture on page 95. Top: ×15,000. Bottom: ×42,000. (Photographs courtesy of Dr. H. Ozawa)

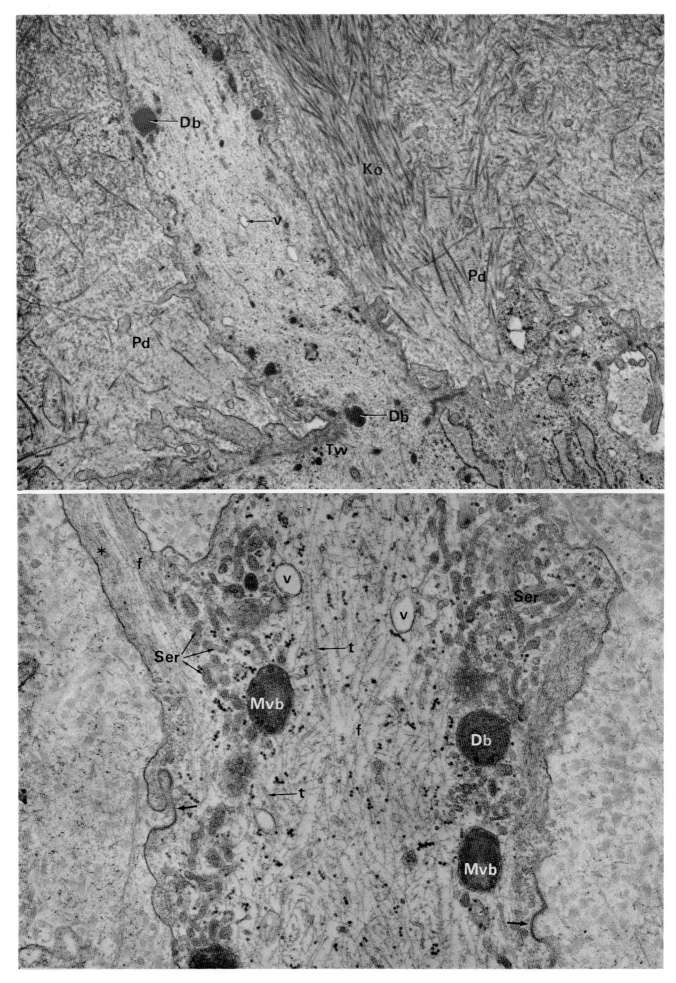

105

Dental pulp

The dental pulp is a richly vascularized and innervated connective tissue contained in the pulp cavity of the tooth.

In the embryonic pulp shown in this picture, the cellular elements are predominant. Most of them are undifferentiated mesenchymal cells of stellate appearance. Their cytoplasm is relatively clear and contains a well-developed Golgi complex (Go), a granular endoplasmic reticulum (Er), a large number of free ribosomes, fine filaments and mitochondria (m). Lipid droplets (Ld) and glycogen particles (Gl) can be seen in some cytoplasm. Their nucleus (N) has one or more large, prominent nucleoli (Nu). The extracellular space is wide and, unlike that in the stellate reticulum of the enamel organ, mostly filled with fine filamentous materials ranging between 100 to 120Å in diameter. They correspond to the argylophilic substance in light microscopy. Between them, collagenous fibrils (Cf) ranging from 400 to 700Å in diameter are also observed. They occasionally appear singly, but more often form small bundles of fibrils.

c: Centriole.
Cap: Blood capillary.

Material and method are the same as those of the pictures on page 95. ×6,500. (Photograph courtesy of Dr. H. Ozawa)

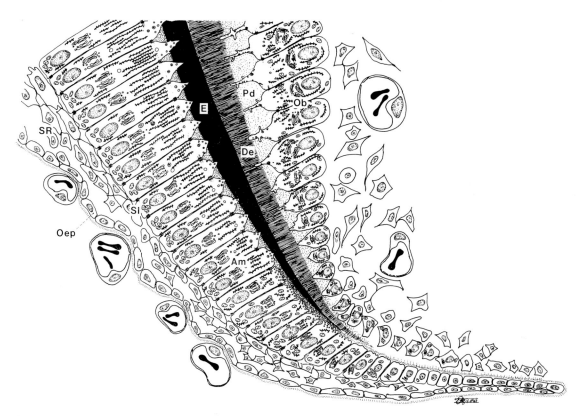

A schematic drawing of a tooth germ at the maturation stage of amelogenesis: In this stage, the enamel organ consists of four types of cell layers: outer enamel epithelium (Oep), stellate reticulum (SR), stratum intermedium (SI), and ameloblastic layer (Am). The enamel (E) is formed by the ameloblasts which are extremely tall, narrow cells with slender cytoplasmic processes called Tomes' processes. On the other hand, the dentin is formed by the odontoblasts (Ob) which are rather stout elongated cells with prominent apical projections called Tomes' fibers. The latter extend throughout the entire width of the dentin, *i. e.* the unmineralized predentin (Pd), and the mineralized dentin (De). (Courtesy of Dr. T. Yajima)

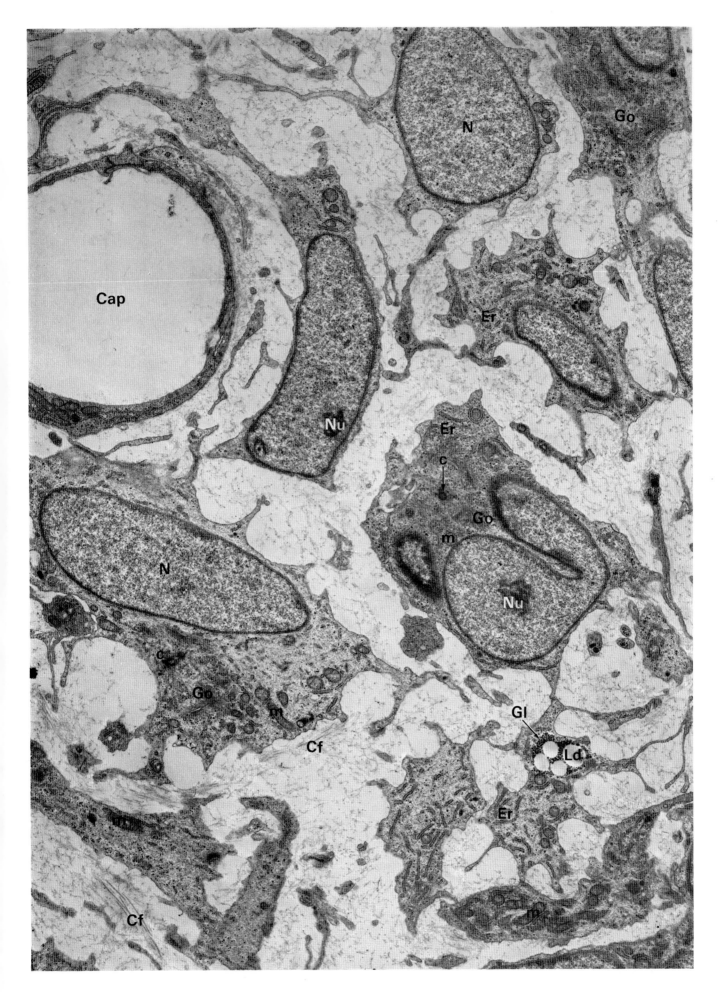

Gastric surface epithelium

The gastric cavity is lined by an epithelium made up of tall, simple columnar cells. The apical cytoplasm of the epithelial cells is occupied by numbers of mucous granules (g) which, when secreted from the cells, protect the mucosal surface from autodigestion by gastric juice.

The apical surface of the epithelium is provided with a few microvilli. The basal surface is firmly attached to the basal lamina (Bl). A wide intercellular space bounded by the inter-digitating microvillous structure of the cell sides is sealed beneath the luminal surface by junctional complexes (Jc). The nucleus (N) with a prominent nucleolus (Nu) is oval in shape and situated toward the base of the cell. The Golgi complex (Go) is large and located in the supranuclear region. Cisterns of granular endoplasmic reticulum and mitochondria are scattered throughout the cytoplasm.

Lu: Lumen.

Biopsy material obtained from the pyloric antrum of a 51-year-old male. Phosphate-buffered 2.0% glutaraldehyde fixation followed by post-fixation with 1.0% osmium tetroxide solution. Uranyl acetate and lead tartarate staining. ×11,000.

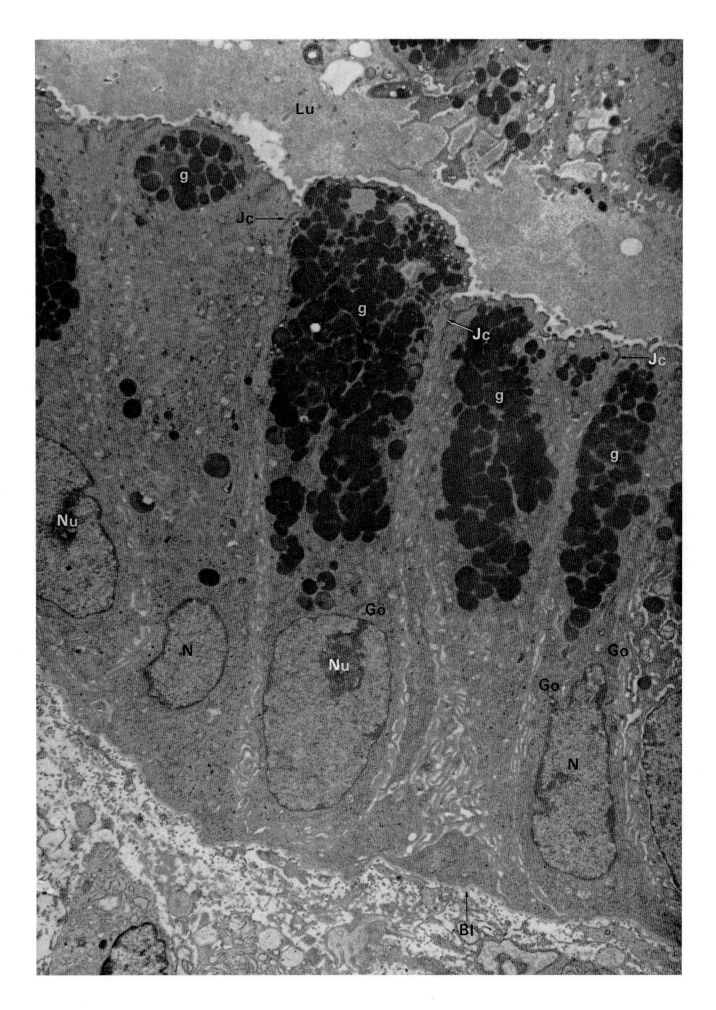

109

Fundic gland

The mucous membrane of the stomach is packed with gastric glands. They are of the simple tubular type with a few branchings. They are classified into three kinds: cardiac, fundic and pyloric. The cardiac and pyloric glands, located in the named regions of the stomach, both secrete mucus. The fundic glands occur in the corpus of the stomach and secrete the gastric juice containing the enzyme pepsin and hydrochloric acid as well as some mucus.

This is a survey electron micrograph showing a cross section of the bottom of a fundic gland. There are parietal cells (Par) with deep intracellular secretory canaliculi (*), chief cells (Cc) having dense granules in their apical cytoplasm, and an endocrine cell (Bg) which is separated from the glandular lumen by a parietal cell covering it.

Cap: Blood capillary.
Glu: Glandular lumen.
Mc: Mast cell.
Pc: Plasma cell.

Gastric corpus of a 48-year-old male. Obtained by biopsy for diagnostic purpose, using a fiber-gastroscope. Phosphate-buffered 2.5% glutaraldehyde fixation followed by post-fixation with 1.0% osmium tetroxide solution. Uranyl acetate and lead tartarate staining. ×4,800.

REFERENCE:

Rubin, W., L. L. Ross, M. H. Sleisenger and G. H. Jeffries: The normal human gastric epithelia. A fine structural study. Lab. Invest., *19*: 598-626, 1968.

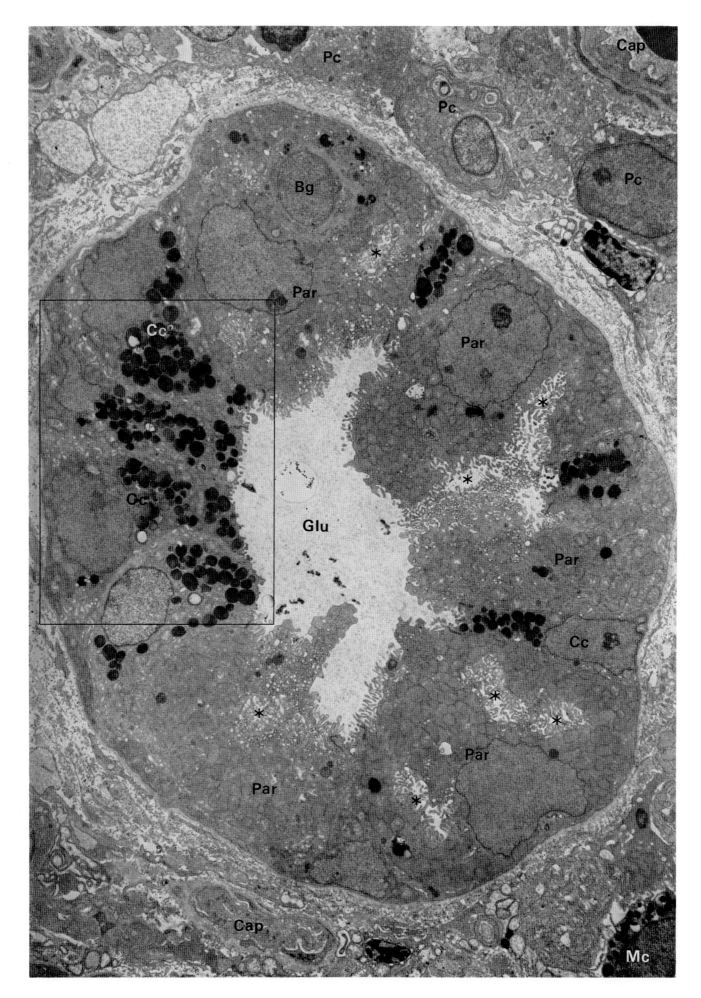

111

Parietal cell

The parietal cells, the acid-secreting cells of the stomach, are located singly or in small groups between other cell types of the fundic gland, especially at the neck portion. They lie on the basal lamina (Bl) with their extensive cell base and contain what seemed to be acidophilic granules in light microscopy, but which turned out to be mitochondria in electron microscopy. The intracellular secretory canaliculi (*), also long known by light microscopists, are projected by numerous microvilli in electron microscopy. Mitochondria (m) filling the cytoplasm are large and ovoid with elaborated cristae mitochondriales. The granular endoplasmic reticulum is scarce and the Golgi complexes (Go) are scattered between the nucleus and the cell base. The cytoplasm near the intracellular secretory canaliculi is filled with small vesicles limited by a smooth membrane sac (arrows). In the bat and some other mammals, the vesicles of the smooth membrane system are said to be tubular in shape and to communicate with the cell surface, but, in man, it remains obscure whether they are vesicular or tubular in shape.

Cc : Chief cell.
Fc : Fibrocyte.
Glu : Glandular lumen.
Jc : Junctional complex.
Ld : Lipid droplet.
Ly : Lysosome.
Nu : Nucleolus.

Material and method are the same as those of the picture on page 111. ×9,500.

REFERENCES:

Ito, S.: The endoplasmic reticulum of gastric parietal cells. J. biophysic. biochem. Cytol., *11*: 333–347, 1961.

Nomura, Y.: On the submicroscopic morphogenesis of parietal cell in the gastric gland of the human fetus. Z. Anat. Entw.-gesch., *125*: 316–356, 1966.

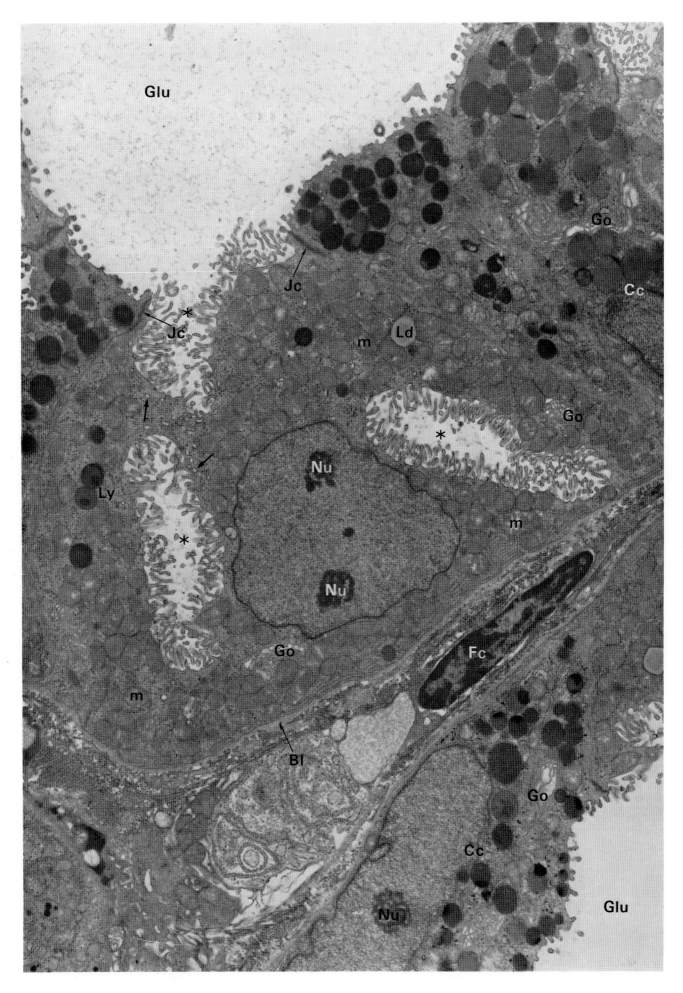

Chief or zymogen cell

The chief cell of the fundic gland secretes pepsinogen, the precursor of pepsin. This cell is situated mainly in the lower part of the fundic gland, is pyramidal in shape and extends from the lumen to the basal lamina (Bl). Its fine structure resembles that of other enzyme-secreting cells such as the pancreatic exocrine cell and the salivary serous cell.

The luminal surface of the chief cell is usually narrow and shows a few apical microvilli. Release of the zymogen granules occurs here. The chief cell attaches to other epithelial cells by junctional complexes (Jc) beneath the luminal surface. The nucleus (N) is spherical in shape, has a prominent nucleolus (Nu) and is located toward the base of the cell. In a starved condition, the apical cytoplasm is filled with dense, round zymogen granules (Zg) which are released when food materials reach the stomach. The Golgi complex (Go) is located in the supranuclear region. The basal cytoplasm is characterized by abundant elements of the granular endoplasmic reticulum, numerous free ribosomes and several mitochondria (m).

Top : This is a higher magnification of the area enclosed by the rectangle in the picture on page 111. There are several chief cells and a part of a parietal cell (Par) in this picture.

Glu : Glandular lumen.

Material and method are the same as those of the picture on page 111.   ×9,500.

Bottom : A basal portion of a chief cell of the fundic gland. Zymogen granules (Zg), mitochondria (m), parallel-arranged cisterns of granular endoplasmic reticulum (Er) and numerous free ribosomes are shown. The outer nuclear membrane is also studded with numerous ribosomes. The basal surface of the cell is smooth and rests on the basal lamina (Bl).

N : Nucleus.

∗ : Cell boundary.

Gastric fundic mucosa of a 58-year-old male. Method for specimen preparation is the same as that of the picture on page 111.   ×26,000.

REFERENCE:

LILLIBRIDGE, C. B.: Membranes of the human pepsinogen granules. J. biophysic. biochem. Cytol., *10*: 145-149, 1961.

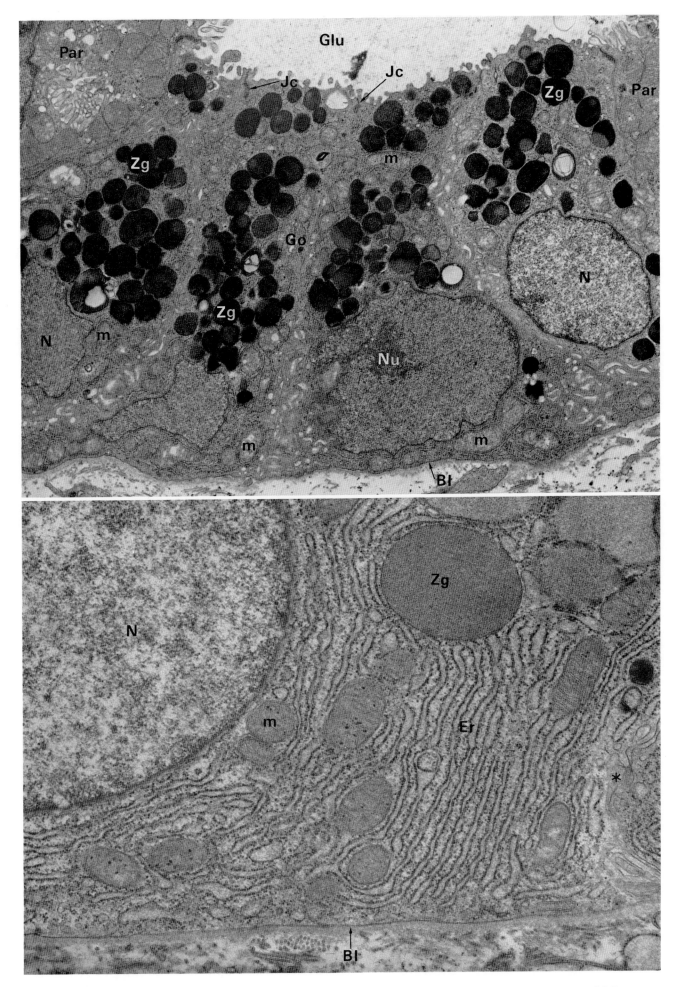

Mucous cell of the pyloric gland (Top)

The pyloric gland is a tubulo-alveolar gland in the lamina propria of the pylorus, and its secretory cells contain mucous granules (Mg) in their apical cytoplasm. Their nuclei, with prominent nucleoli (Nu), are flattened against the basal lamina (Bl). Golgi complexes (Go) are well developed and are multifocally situated in the supra- and para-nuclear regions. Small mitochondria (m) and cisterns of granular endoplasmic reticulum are scattered throughout the cytoplasm.

> Glu: Glandular lumen.

Pyloric antrum of a 61-year-old male with gastric ulcer. Method for specimen preparation is the same as that of the picture on page 109. ×6,000.

Probable gastrin-secreting cell (Bottom)

The pyloric gland contains, together with mucus-secreting cells, many endocrine cells with basal granules (g) consisting of a loose and irregular core and a round sac. The cell apex reaches the lumen (Glu) and is provided with some microvilli (Mv). This type cell, generally called G cell, is now believed to secrete gastrin, the hormone which promotes gastric acid secretion.

> Bl: Basal lamina.
> c: Centriole.
> Er: Granular endoplasmic reticulum.
> Go: Golgi complex.
> Ly: Lysosome.
> Mg: Mucous granule.
> N: Nucleus.

Material and method are the same as those of the top picture. ×9,500. (Arch. histol. jap., *32*: 277, 1970)

REFERENCES:

KOBAYASHI, S., T. FUJITA and T. SASAGAWA: Electron microscope studies on the endocrine cells of the human gastric fundus. Arch. histol. jap., *32*: 429–444, 1971.

PEARSE, A. G. E., I. COULLING, B. WEAVERS and S. FRIESEN: The endocrine polypeptide cells of the human stomach, duodenum, and jejunum. Gut, *11*: 649–658, 1970.

SASAGAWA, T., S. KOBAYASHI and T. FUJITA: The endocrine cells in the human pyloric antrum. An electron microscope study of biopsy materials. Arch. histol. jap., *32*: 275–288, 1970.

SOLCIA, E., C. CAPELLA and G. VASSALLO: Endocrine cells of the stomach and pancreas in states of gastric hypersecretion. Rendic. R. Gastroenterol., *2*: 147–158, 1970.

SOLCIA, E., G. VASSALLO and C. CAPELLA: Studies on the G cells of the pyloric mucosa, the probable site of gastrin secretion. Gut, *10*: 379–388, 1969.

SOLCIA, E., G. VASSALLO and C. CAPELLA: Cytology and cytochemistry of hormone producing cells of the upper gastrointestinal tract. In: W. CREUTZFELDT (ed.): Origin, chemistry, physiology and Pathophysiology of the Gastrointestinal Hormones, Schattauer Verlag, Stuttgart, 1970. (p. 3–29).

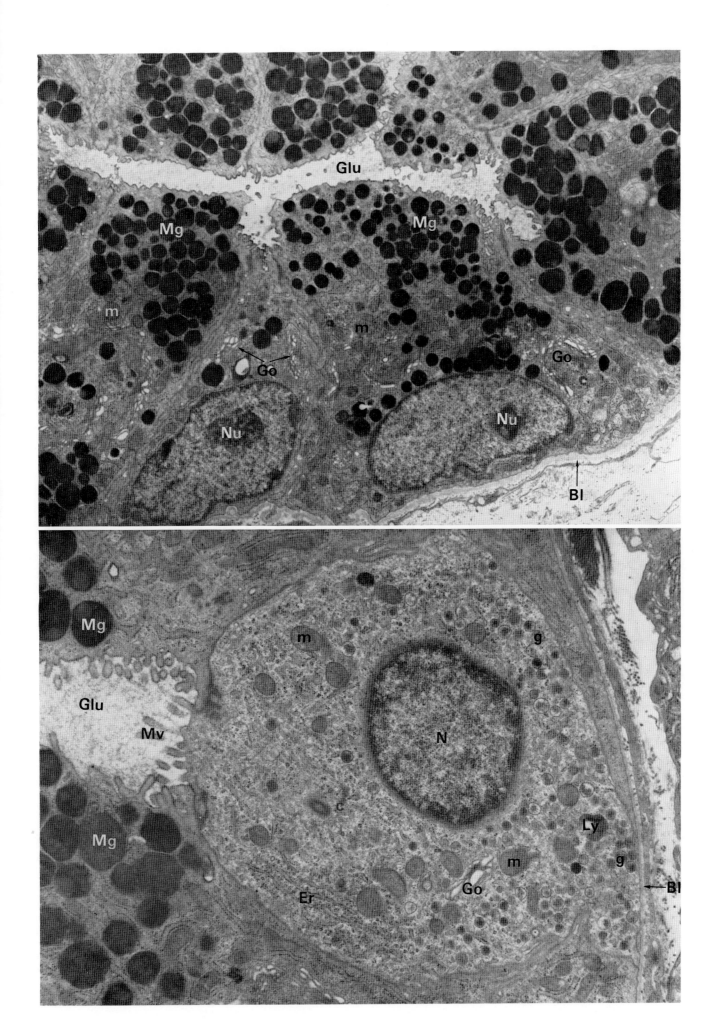

Epithelium covering the tip of the intestinal villus (Top)

The tip of the intestinal villus is the site where various nutrients are most actively absorbed. The luminal surface of the columnar absorptive cells is covered by a prominent striated border (Stb) which consists of an accumulation of microvilli. The basal surface of the cells is firmly attached to the basal lamina (Bl). The intercellular space is greatly distended and occupied by a granular substance of low electron opacity and several emigrating lymphocytes (Lc). The luminal end of the intercellular space is sealed with a junctional complex (Jc). All nutrients are thus absorbed through the cytoplasm of the columnar cells.

The columnar absorptive cells of the small intestine are continually exfoliated and are replaced by cells that arise from mitotic activity in the deep portion of the intestinal crypt.

Ilu : Intestinal lumen.
N : Nucleus of the columnar absorptive cell.
R : Erythrocyte in the capillary lumen.

Epithelium covering the trunk of the villus (Bottom)

The absorptive function of the trunk of the villus is not so active as that of the tip of the villus.

In this picture there are columnar absorptive cells with a striated border (Stb), two goblet cells (Gob) and an endocrine cell (Ec). The intercellular space is narrow and contains a migrating lymphocyte (Lc). The epithelium is deeply indented at the orifices of the goblet cells (arrows).

Cap : Blood capillary.

Top and Botton: Duodenum of a 68-year-old female with gastric cancer. Obtained by operation. Phosphate-buffered 2.5% glutaraldehyde fixation followed by 1.3% osmium tetroxide post-fixation. Uranyl acetate and lead tartarate staining. Top and Bottom: ×2,500.

REFERENCE:

Trier, J. S.: Morphology of the epithelium of the small intestine. Handbook of physiology: Alimentary canal, Vol. 3. Washington, D. C.: American Physiological Society, 1968. (p. 1125–1175).

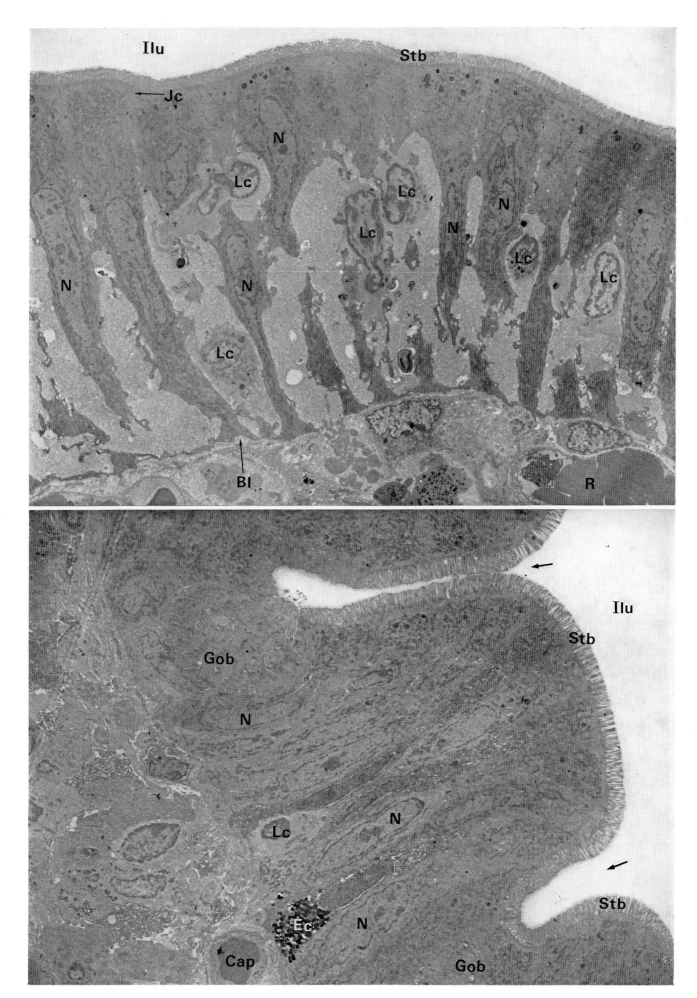

Columnar cell and goblet cell in the small intestinal epithelium

In this micrograph are seen several columnar cells and a goblet cell.

The luminal surface of the columnar cell is covered by a striated border (Stb) consisting of a large number of microvilli. This is a structural device for increasing the area of the luminal surface of the cell through which nutrients are absorbed. The neighboring cells are tightly attached to each other by a junctional complex (Jc) beneath their free surface. The lateral surface of the cells is irregular in contour due to interdigitating cytoplasmic processes (∗). The basal cell surface is relatively smooth and rests on the basal lamina (Bl).

The nucleus (N) of the columnar absorptive cell is usually oval in shape and is located below the middle of the cell. It contains one or more prominent nucleoli (Nu). The cytoplasm subjacent to the striated border appears to contain only a filamentous material and a few small vesicles and is called "terminal web" (Tw). Mitochondria (m) and cisterns of granular endoplasmic reticulum are found dispersed throughout the cytoplasm, but not in the terminal web. Golgi complexes (Go) are located in the supranuclear region.

A goblet cell (Gob) is located between the columnar absorptive cells. It is characterized by an accumulation of large round granules (g) in the apical cytoplasm. These granules correspond to the PAS positive granules seen in light microscopy and are known to contain certain mucoproteins. The Golgi complexes (Go) are exceedingly well-developed in this kind of cell. Lamellated cisterns of the Golgi complex, which is located in the supranuclear region, surround accumulations of secretory granules. Numerous mitochondria and parallel-arranged cisterns of granular endoplasmic reticulum are scattered in the para- and infra-nuclear regions.

Ilu: Intestinal lumen.

Ly: Lysosome.

Jejunum of a 35-year-old female of protein-loosing syndrome. Biopsy material obtained for diagnostic purpose, using a fiber-enterosope. Phosphate-buffered 2.0% osmium tetroxide fixation. Lead tartarate staining. ×5,000.

REFERENCES:

HARTMAN, R. E., R. B. W. SMITH, R. S. HARTMAN, C. E. BUTTERWORTH and J. M. MOLEWORTH: The electron microscopy of human intestinal epithelium obtained with the Crosby intestinal biopsy capsule. J. biophysic. biochem. Cytol., 5: 171–172, 1959.

LADMAN, A. J., H. A. PADYKULA and E. W. STRAUSS: A morphological study of fat transport in the normal human jejunum. Amer. J. Anat., 112: 389–419, 1963.

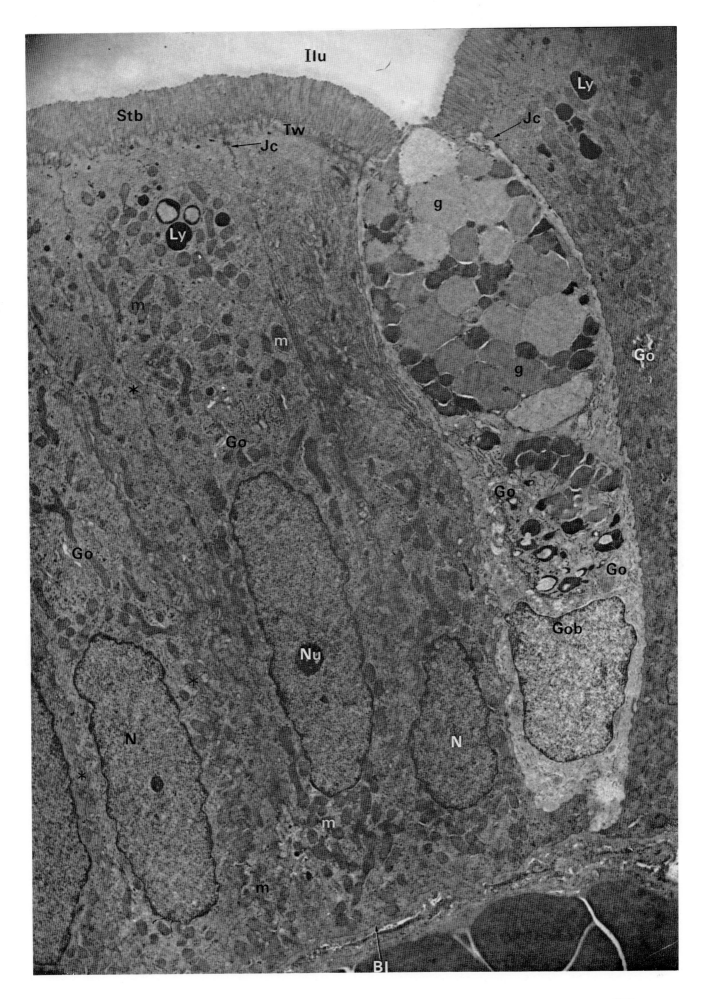

INTESTINE

Striated border

Each columnar absorptive cell of the small intestine is said to bear more than a thousand microvilli. They greatly enlarge the surface area of the cell to facilitate the absorption of nutrient materials. They are uniform in length and thickness and form a striated border.

Each microvillus is limited by a plasma membrane which shows a distinct trilamellar structure. The cytoplasm within the microvillus contains longitudinally-arranged bundles of thin fibrils which seem to end on the inner aspect of the plasma membrane at the apex of the microvillus (see the bottom left picture). These fibrils extend downward from the microvilli into the area subjacent to the free surface. This area, called terminal web (Tw), is devoid of the usual cell organelles. A fuzzy surface coat covers the free surface of the microvilli. It is an extracellular layer of a polysaccharide-rich material and is believed to play an important role in the absorption of nutrients.

The columnar absorptive cells are firmly attached near the luminal surface by a typical junctional complex consisting of a tight junction (Zo), an intermediate junction (Za) and a desmosome (Ma). The detail of the junctional complex will be shown in the micrograph on page 125.

Top left : A transverse section of the striated border and the apex of epithelial cells.

Jejunum of a 35-year-old female with protein-loosing syndrome. Biopsy material obtained for diagnostic purpose, using a fiber-enteroscope. Phosphate-buffered 2.0% osmium tetroxide fixation. Lead tartarate staining. ×43,000.

Top right : A cross section of the striated border and the apex of two adjacent epithelial cells showing cross sections of microvilli and the zonula occludens of junctional complex.

Duodenum of a 68-year-old female with gastric cancer. Obtained by operation. Phosphate-buffered 2.5% glutaraldehyde fixation followed by post-fixation with 1.0% osmium tetroxide solution. Uranyl acetate and lead tartarate staining. ×43,000.

Bottom left : Longitudinal section of the tips of microvilli.

Bottom right : A cross section of microvilli and a portion of terminal web (Tw) of a columnar absorptive cell.

Bottom left and right: Duodenum of a 56-year-old male with cholecystitis. Biopsy material obtained during surgical operation. Phosphate-buffered 2.5% glutaraldehyde fixation followed by post-fixation with 1.0% osmium tetroxide solution. Uranyl acetate and lead citrate staining. Bottom left and right: ×131,000. (Photographs courtesy of Dr. H. OZAWA)

REFERENCES:

BROWN, A. L.: Microvilli of the human jejunal epithelial cell. J. Cell Biol., *13*: 623–627, 1962.
LAGUENS, R. and M. BRIONES: Fine structure of the microvillus of columnar epithelium cells of human intestine. Lab. Invest., *14*: 1616–1623, 1965.

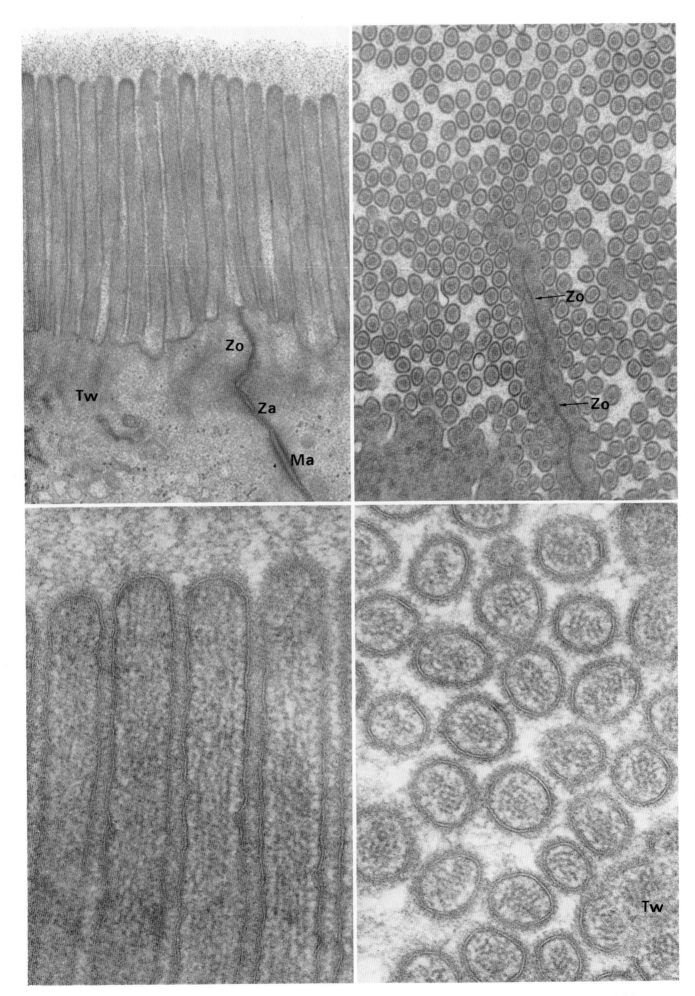

Junctional complex between two columnar cells

The epithelial cells generally are tightly connected in their subapical level by a device which light microscopists call terminal bar, so that the intercellular spaces are closed against the epithelial free surface. The terminal bar corresponds to the junctional complex in electron microscopy and is known to consist of three different parts. A tight junction (zonula occludens) characterized by the fusion of plasma membranes occurs immediately beneath the lumen. Then follow an intermediate junction (zonula adherens) and a desmosome (macula adherens).

Af : Anchoring filaments extending from the core of microvilli to the terminal web. Some fibrils insert themselves into the intermediate junction.

Ilu : Intestinal lumen.

Ma : Desmosome (macula adherens) in which the intercellular material (arrow) is prominent.

Tw : Terminal web.

Za : Intermediate junction (zonula adherens) extending from c to d.

Zo : Tight junction (zonula occludens) which occupies the regions between a and b.

From the duodenum of a 68-year-old female with gastric cancer. Obtained by operation. Phosphate-buffered 2.5% glutaraldehyde fixation followed by 1.3% osmium tetroxide post-fixation. Uranyl acetate and lead citrate staining. ×182,000. (Photograph courtesy of Dr. H. OZAWA)

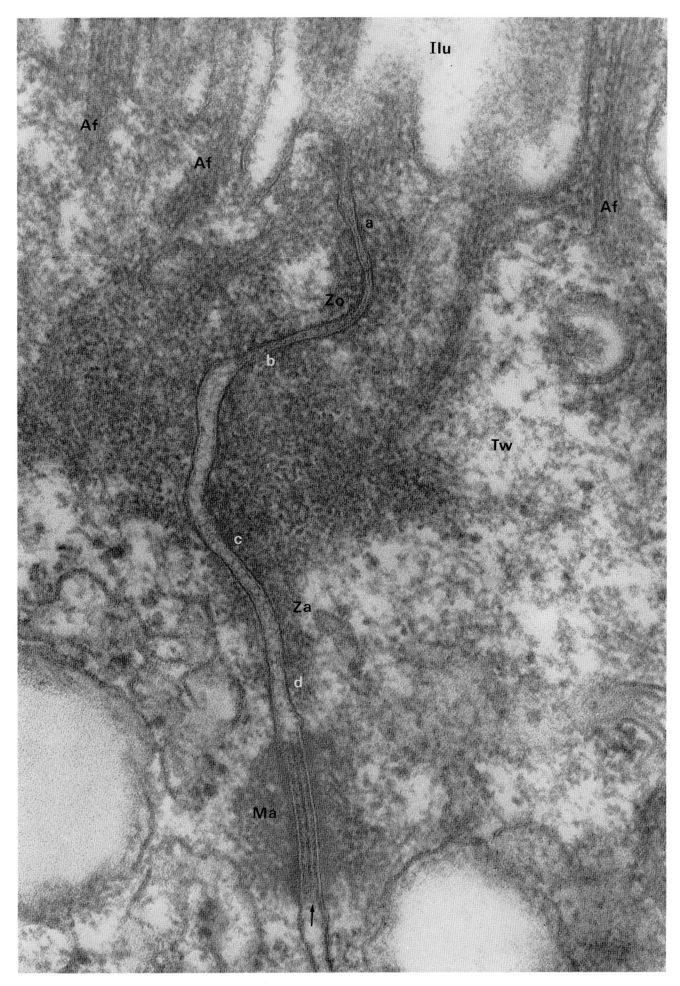

Intestinal crypt (crypt of Lieberkühn) (Top)

The intestinal crypt is a simple tubular gland seen in the mucous membrane of the small and the large intestine. Its wall consists of a simple columnar epithelium containing, in the small intestine, four types of cells: columnar, goblet, endocrine and Paneth cells. The crypt of the large intestine is characterized by an abundance of goblet cells and an absence of Paneth cells.

In this picture is shown a portion of an intestinal crypt in the duodenum. There are columnar cells with relatively loose microvilli on their luminal surface, goblet cells (Gob) filled with numerous mucous granules and two endocrine cells of different morphological features. The cell on the left (Bg II), which reaches the lumen, contains large, round basal granules, whereas the right cell (Bg III), which does not reach the lumen (Lu) in this section, has much smaller granules.

In the center of this picture, a mitotic figure (Mi) in a columnar cell is seen. The columnar cells in the intestinal crypt are undifferentiated absorptive cells which later pass up to the villus to be shed from the tip of the villus.

Bl : Basal lamina.
Cap : Capillary.

Duodenum of a 59-year-old male with gastric cancer. Obtained by operation. Phosphate-buffered glutaraldehyde fixation followed by post-fixation with 1.0% osmium tetroxide solution. Stained with uranyl acetate and lead tartarate solution. ×4,000.

Paneth cell (Bottom)

Paneth cells are seen in the fundus of the intestinal crypt of the small intestine. They resemble in fine structure the pancreatic exocrine cells which produce digestive enzymes. Their apical cytoplasm is filled with large round granules which are stained with eosin in light microscopy. These granules contain abundant mucopolysaccaride and arginine-rich proteins and show the activities of peptidase and lysozyme. The cytoplasm, especially in the cell base, is filled with cisterns of granular endoplasmic reticulum (Er).

c : Centriole
Lc : Migrating lymphocyte.
m : Mitochondrion.
Nu : Nucleolus.

Duodenum of a 68-year-old female with gastric cancer. Obtained by operation. Method for specimen preparation is the same as those of the top picture. ×7,500.

REFERENCES :

KOBAYASHI, S., T. FUJITA and T. SASAGAWA : The endocrine cells of human duodenal mucosa. An electron microscope study. Arch. histol. jap., *31* : 477–494, 1970.

TRIER, J.S. : Studies on small intestinal crypt epithelium. I. The fine structure of the crypt epithelium of the proximal small intestine of fasting humans. J. Cell Biol., *18* : 599–620, 1963.

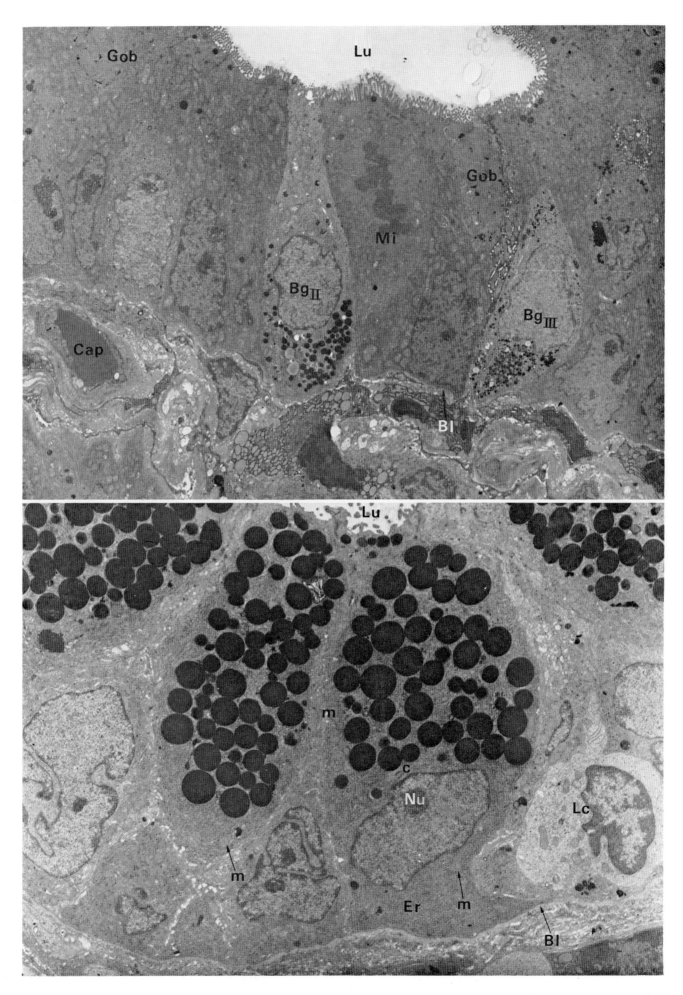

Endocrine cell of an open type (Top)

The gastro-enteric endocrine cells are classified into an open and a closed type. The open type cell is pyramidal in shape and reaches the lumen (Lu) with its apical process. It has been suggested that with its apical process this type of endocrine cell may perceive chemical information of the lumen and be able to control the granule release from the basal surface of the cell. On the other hand, the closed type endocrine cell which occurs in the gastric fundus and the rectum is flattened in shape and isolated from the lumen by other cells covering it. It may receive physical stimuli such as pressure, temperature and tension of the intestinal lumen.

This micrograph shows an open type endocrine cell found in the crypt of the duodenum. The luminal surface of the tapered cell process bears a tuft of microvilli (Mv). The basal cytoplasm is crowded with round secretory granules of high electron opacity bounded by a single limiting membrane. Sets of Golgi complexes (Go) are located at the supranuclear region. Small, dense granules seen in the Golgi complexes (arrows) may suggest the formation of the basal granules in these regions. Parallel-arranged cisterns of granular endoplasmic reticulum (Er) are seen around the nucleus. The hormone that this type of cell might produce is unidentified as yet.

- Bl : Basal lamina.
- Jc : Junctional complex.
- m : Mitochondrion.
- Mg : Mucous granule.
- Nu : Nucleolus.
- Ygc : Young goblet cell.

From the duodenum of a 59-year-old male with gastric cancer. Obtained by surgical operation. Phosphate-buffered 2.5% glutaraldehyde fixation followed by post-fixation with 1.0% osmium tetroxide solution. ×13,000.

Duodenal gland of Brunner (Bottom)

The duodenal gland of Brunner is a branched and coiled tubular gland in the tunica sub-mucosa of the first part of the duodenum near the pylorus. The terminal portion of the gland secretes an alkaline mucin which enters the intestinal lumen through the duct which opens into the intestinal crypt.

In this micrograph, parts of two terminal portions are shown. They are separated by a connective tissue containing bundles of collagenous fibrils (Cf), fibrocytes (Fc) and profiles of blood capillaries (Cap). The glandular cells are characterized by an accumulation of mucous granules (Mg) of medium electron opacity in the apical cytoplasm. The nucleus (N) with prominent nucleoli is located at the base of the cell. Golgi complexes (Go) and granular endoplasmic reticulum are well developed around the nucleus.

- Glu : Glandular lumen.
- Ly : Lysosome.

From the duodenum of a 68-year-old female with gastric cancer. Obtained by operation. Method for specimen preparation is the same as that of the top picture. ×3,300.

REFERENCE:

Leeson, T. S. and C. R. Leeson: The fine structure of Brunner's glands in man. J. Anat., *103*: 263-276, 1968.

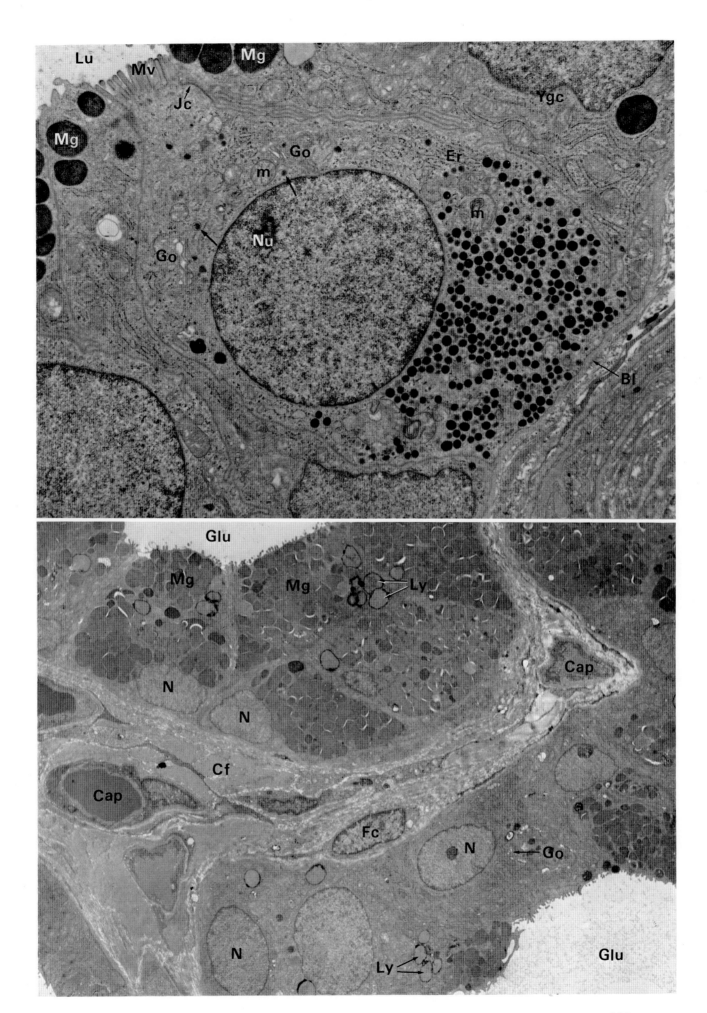

129

Endocrine cell of the intestinal crypt

In this micrograph is shown a deep portion of a crypt of Lieberkühn. There are several endocrine cells: two cells (EC) with dense polymorphous basal granules, a cell (L) with large round granules and two cells (D) whose granules appear identical with those of the D cells in the pancreatic islet. Although their luminal protrusions are not seen in this picture, it is highly probable that every endocrine cell seen in this micrograph opens onto the lumen at different levels of the section.

Bl: Basal lamina.
Cap: Capillary.
f: Bundles of cytoplasmic filaments.
Go: Golgi complex.
Lu: Lumen.

From the duodenum of a 59-year-old male with gastric cancer. Method is the same as that of the top picture on page 129. ×7,000. (Arch. histol. jap., *31*: 480, 1970)

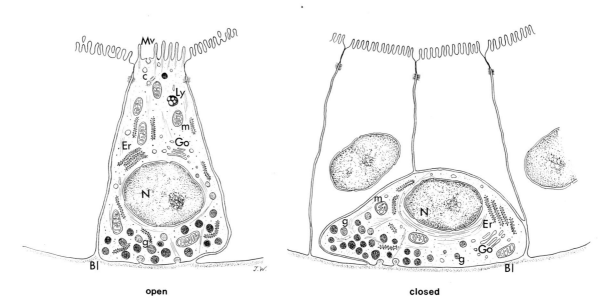

open   **closed**

Diagram showing two types of gastro-enteric endocrine cells
Bl: Basal lamina. c: Centriole. Er: Granular endoplasmic reticulum. g: Secretory granule. Go: Golgi complex. Ly: Lysosome. m: Mitochondrion. Mv: Microvillus. N: Nucleus.

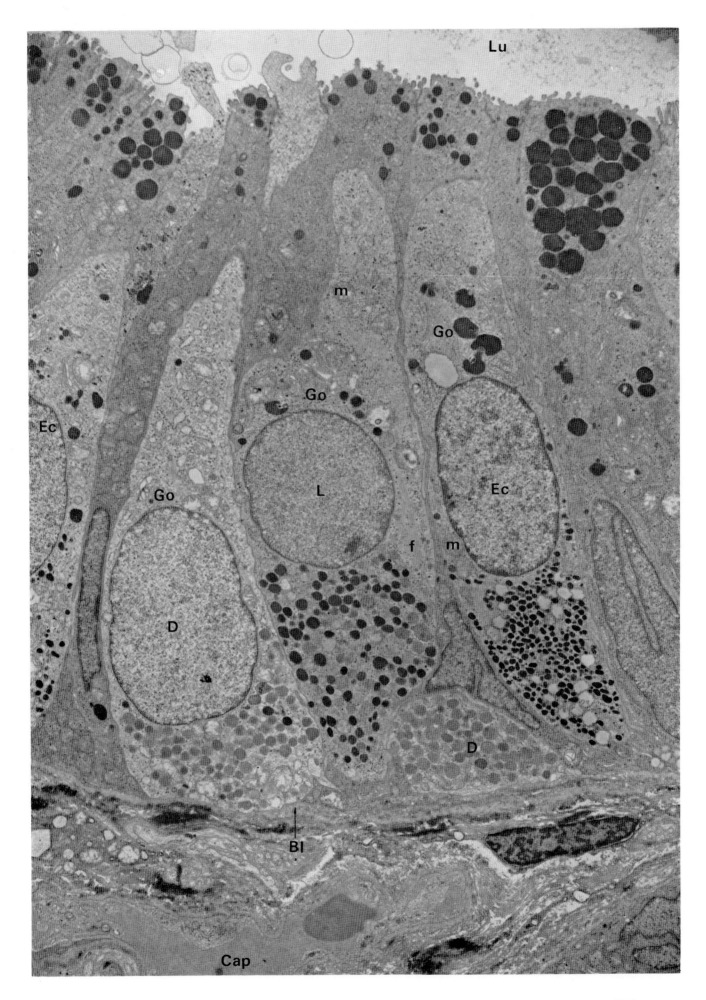

Surface epithelium of the large intestine

The main function of the large intestine is the absorption of water. It can also absorb food nutrients to a limited extent. Its lining consists of a simple columnar epithelium containing columnar absorptive cells and goblet cells (Gob). The goblet cells are much more numerous in the large intestine than in the small intestine.

The columnar absorptive cells of the large intestine, unlike those of the small intestine, have no distinct striated border on their luminal surfaces, though several microvilli (Mv) are found on their luminal surfaces. In the lower half of the epithelium, the intercellular space is widely distended and the lateral surfaces of the cells show complex plications. The wide intercellular space is thought to facilitate the absorption of water. Small round bodies (arrows) seen in the cytoplasm beneath the free surface are known to contain acid phosphatase and other hydrolytic enzymes, and are called apical granules or apical lysosomes.

The fine structure of the goblet cell (Gob) shown in this picture essentially corresponds to that in the small intestine shown in the picture on page 121. However, the mucous granules (g) in this micrograph, which was obtained after successive fixation in glutaraldehyde and osmium tetroxide, appear denser than in the picture on page 121, which was obtained after single fixation in osmium tetroxide.

Bl : Basal lamina.
Go : Golgi complex.
m : Mitochondrion.
Mv : Microvillus.
N : Nucleus.
Nu : Nucleolus.

Transverse colon of a 28-year-old male. Obtained by anal biopsy for diagnostic purpose, using a fiber-colonoscope. Phosphate-buffered 2.5% glutaraldehyde fixation followed by 1.0% osmium tetroxide post-fixation. Uranyl acetate and lead tartarate staining. ×7,000.

REFERENCES:

Osaka, M., T. Sasagawa, S. Kobayashi and T. Fujita: The endocrine cells in the human colon and rectum. An electron microscope study of biopsy materials. Arch. histol. jap., *33*: 247–260, 1971.

Pittman, F. E. and J. C. Pittman: An electron microscopic study of the epithelium of normal human sigmoid colonic mucosa. Gut, *7*: 644–661, 1966.

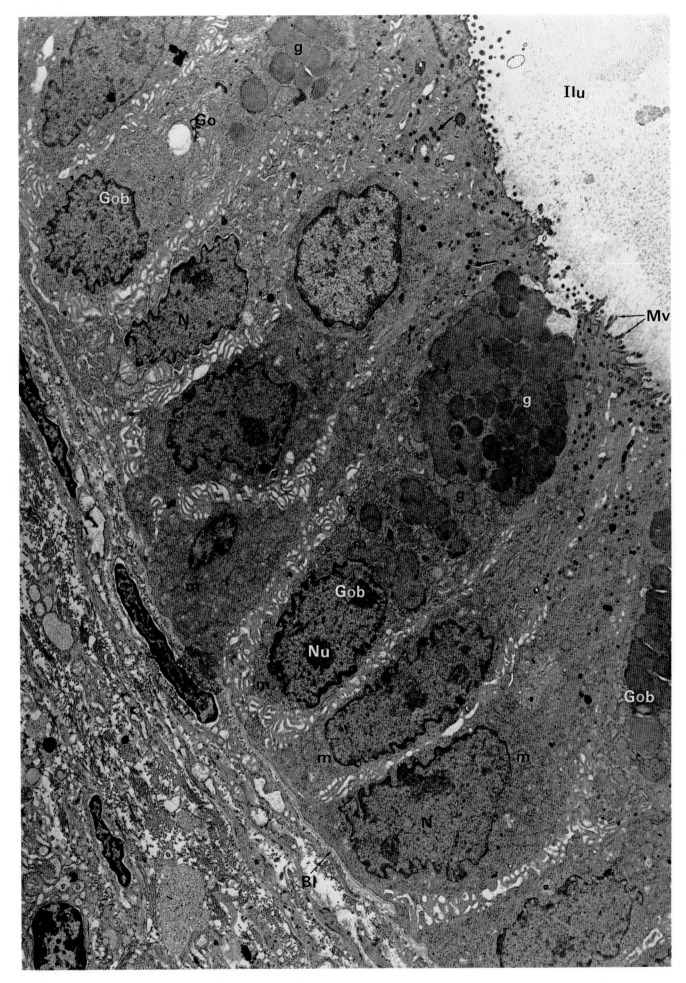

Parenchyme of the liver

The liver is the largest digestive gland of the body. It secretes bile and is also of great importance in both carbohydrate and protein metabolism. Its parenchyme consists of a continuous mass of liver cells perforated by a network of tunnels in which the sinusoids run.

This micrograph shows a peripheral portion of a liver lobule. The liver cells are polyhedral in shape and have one or, occasionally, two nuclei (N) in their center. Mitochondria (m), glycogen particles (Gl) profiles of granular endoplasmic reticulum (Er) are scattered within the cytoplasm. A few lipofuscin pigments (Lp), dense bodies (Db) and lipid droplets (Ld) are also contained there. Bile capillaries (Bc) are seen as clear intercellular spaces between adjacent cells. One of the sinusoidal capillaries (Sin) which irrigate the hepatic lobule is cross cut at the lower part of this micrograph. In the upper left corner an interlobular connective tissue (Ict) containing a vein is seen.

    Ed :   Endothetial cell of interlobular vein.
    Jc :   Junctional complex.
    Nu :   Nucleolus
    R :   Erythrocyte.
    Va :   Vacuole of unknown nature.

Liver of a 39-year-old female patient with cholelithiasis (silent stone). Obtained by surgical operation. Fixation in 2.0% glutaraldehyde followed by post-fixation in 2.0% osmium tetroxide in phosphate buffer. Uranyl acetate and lead tartarate staining. ×3,500.

REFERENCES:

Brown, D. B., J. Delor, M. Greider and W. J. Frajola : The electron microscopy of human liver. Gastroenterol., *32*: 103–118, 1957.

Cossel, L, : Die menschliche Leber im Electronenmikroskop. Gustav Fischer, Jena, 1964.

Tanikawa, K. : Ultrastructural aspects of the liver and its disorders. Igaku Shoin Ltd., Tokyo, 1968.

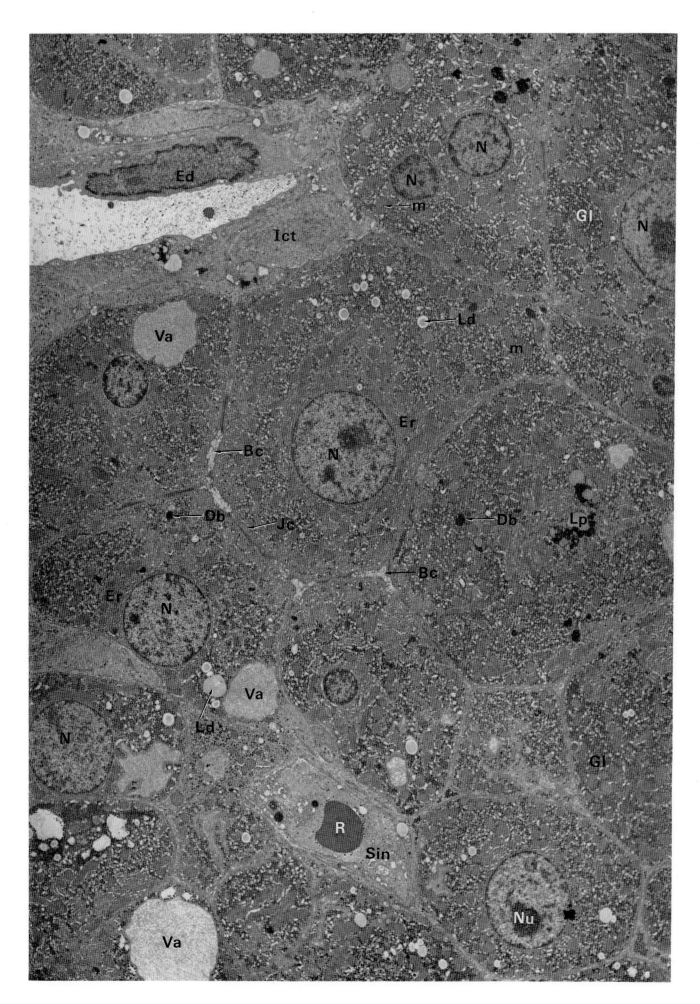

Liver cell

The liver cell subserves several important functions. It takes up blood-glucose and stores it as a form of glycogen to maintain the blood-glucose concentration. It is important in the maintenance of lipid levels in circulating blood. Lipids synthesized from carbohydrate and protein, those from chyromicrons and those released from fat cells are incorporated into lipoproteins and are transported in the blood as occasion demands. It elaborates proteins such as fibrinogen and plasma albumin and also produces urea as a by-product of protein metabolism. In addition, it synthesizes cholesterol, secrets bile salts, and plays an important role in the excretion of bile pigments.

This micrograph shows a portion of a liver cell. The cytoplasm is largely occupied by dilated cisterns of granular endoplasmic reticulum (Er) in which synthesis of proteins occurs. Tubules of smooth-surfaced endoplasmic reticulum are continuous with cisterns of granular endoplasmic reticulum. It is said that some of them are responsible for the elaboration of cholesterol. Glycogen particles (Gl) occur singly (β particles) or in rosettes (α particles). They occupy the interstice between the tubules of smooth-surfaced endoplasmic reticulum. A Golgi complex (Go) consisting of vesicles and cisterns is present in the perinuclear region. Mitochondria (m) are large in size, ovoid in shape, and have only a small number of cristae mitochondriales. Intramitochondrial granules (Img) are somewhat conspicuous. The nucleus is made of karyoplasm surrounded by a nuclear envelope. Heterochromatin (Hc) which appears like a mass of dense particles is mostly located in the peripheral portion of the nucleus. Heterochromatin situated in the circumference of the nucleolus is called nucleolus-associated chromatin (Nac). Tangled strands of nucleolonema (Nm) of the nucleolus are studded with dense granules. Pars amorpha of the nucleolus is not shown in this picture. The nuclear envelope consists of an outer (Om) and an inner membrane (Im) which are separated by a narrow space called perinuclear cistern. These membranes are at places perforated by numerous nuclear pores (arrows) through which the karyoplasm is thought to communicate with the cytoplasm. Note a thin membranous structure which traverses the nuclear pore.

Ec: Euchromatin.

Surgically-obtained liver of a 39-year-old female with cholelithiasis. Phosphate-buffered 2.5% glutaraldehyde fixation followed by 2.0% osmium tetroxide post-fixation. Uranyl acetate and lead tartarate staining. ×48,000.

REFERENCES:

BIEMPICA, L.: Human hepatic microbodies with crystalloid cores. J. Cell Biol., *29*: 383–386, 1966.
ESSNER, E. and A. B. NOVIKOFF: Human hepatocellular pigments and lysosomes. J. Ultrastr. Res., *3*: 374–391, 1960.

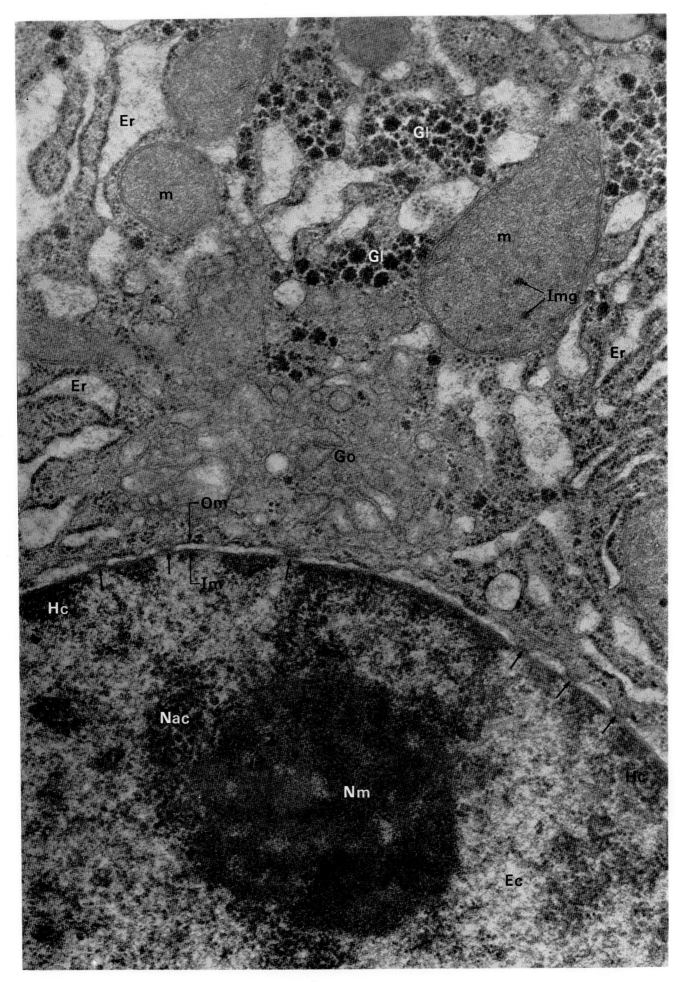

137

Hepatic sinusoid and Kupffer cell (Top)

The hepatic sinusoid is a special type of blood capillary running between the liver cell plates to be gathered into the central vein. Its lining cells are composed of two types: endothelial cell and Kupffer cell. The endothelial cell (Ed) is attenuated and has no marked projections on its free surface. The Kupffer cell (Kc) is larger in size than the former, and possesses numerous long cytoplasmic processes extending from the cell surface. This cell is characterized by abundant lysosomes (Ly) and well-developed Golgi complexes (Go). It has an ability to phagocytise particulate matters such as bacteria and erythrocytes. There is much argument as yet as to whether this cell is originated from the sinusoid endothelial cell.

The hepatic sinusoid is separated from the liver cell by a narrow space (Ds) called space of Disse. This contains numerous microvilli (Mv) projected from the liver cell (Lc) and bundles of collagenous fibrils (Cf) which correspond to reticular fibers of light microscopy.

m : Mitochondrion.
N : Nucleus.
Nu : Nucleolus.
Pl : Blood platelet.
Slu : Sinusoid lumen.

Fat-storing cell (Bottom)

In the space of Disse, a special type of cell containing fat droplets (Fd) is occasionally found. This cell called fat-storing cell of Ito (Fsc) is thought to be derived from a fibroblastic cell. Vitamin A of the liver is mostly kept in the fat droplets of this cell.

The liver cell (Lc) in this micrograph contains many microbodies (Mb), which are characteristic of liver cells and of the proximal tubule cells of the kidney, and contain the enzymes such as peroxidase and D-amino acid oxidase.

Top and Bottom: Surgically-obtained liver of 61-year-old male with esophageal cancer. Phosphate-buffered 2.0% glutaraldehyde fixation followed by 2.0% osmium tetroxide post fixation. Uranyl acetate and lead tartarate staining. Top and Bottom: ×10,000.

REFERENCE:

ITO, T. and S. SHIBASAKI: Electron microscopic study on the hepatic sinusoidal wall and the fat-storing cells in the normal human liver. Arch. histol. jap., *29*: 137-192, 1968.

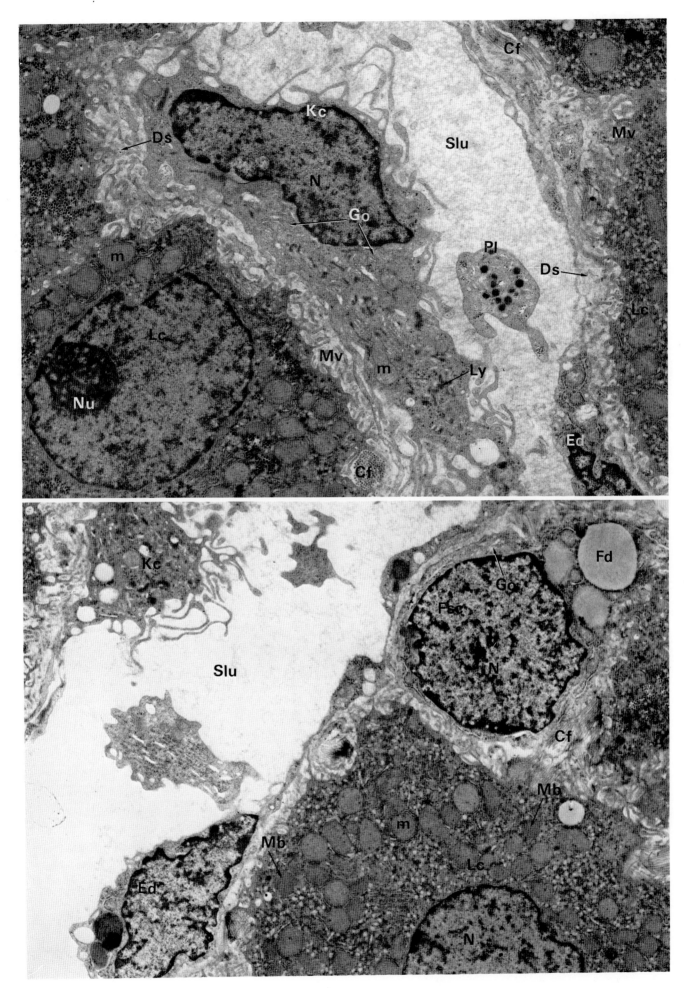

Bile capillary (Top)

The bile capillary is formed between two or three adjacent liver cells. Its narrow lumen (Blu) is bordered by cell membranes of the liver cells which are closely attached to each other by junctional complexes (Jc). Several microvilli (Mv) project from the liver cells into the lumen. Golgi complexes (Go) are usually located in the cytoplasm near the bile capillary.

Er : Granular endoplasmic reticulum.
Gl : Glycogen particles.
Ly : Lysosome.
m : Mitochondrion.

Transitional portion from the bile capillary to the small bile duct (Bottom)

The bile capillary is connected with the small bile duct at the peripheral portion of the hepatic lobule. Here, the liver cells (Lc) forming the bile capillary are replaced by the epithelial cells of the bile duct (Bep), which are cuboidal in shape and smaller in size than the liver cells. The liver cell and the bile duct epithelial cell are closely attached by junctional complexes (Jc). A portion of the interlobular connective tissue is seen in the lower right corner.

Bl : Basal lamina.
Ly : Lysosome.
N : Nucleus.

Top and Bottom : Liver of a 52-year-old male clinically diagnosed as hyperlipemia. Obtained by a needle biopsy for diagnostic purpose. Phosphate-buffered 2.0% glutaraldehyde fixation followed by 2.0% osmium tetroxide post fixation. Lead tartarate staining. Top : ×30,000. Bottom : ×10,000.

REFERENCE:

Biava, C. G.: Studies on cholestasis. A re-evaluation of the fine structure of normal human bile canaliculi. Lab. Invest., *13*: 840–864, 1964.

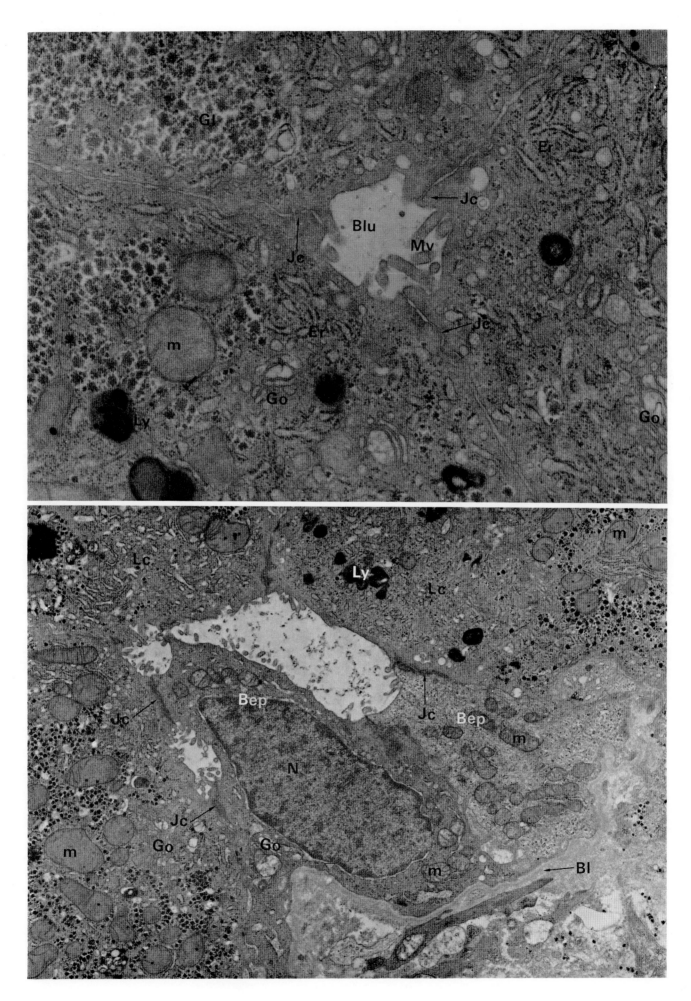

141

Interlobular portal area

The interlobular portal areas are islands of connective tissue at corners of each liver lobule. They are continuous with the superficial covering of the liver and contain the so-called " portal triad " consisting of the hepatic artery, portal vein and bile duct as these ramify within the liver.

In this micrograph a portion of a portal area containing an interlobular vein, which is a branch of the portal vein, and a small bile duct is shown. The vein is lined by a thin sheet of endothelium (Ed) surrounded by a few smooth muscle cells (Sm). The bile duct is composed of cuboidal cells with small nuclei (N) which are similar to those in other conducting ducts. Their cytoplasm contains a small number of cell organelles such as mitochondria (m), Golgi complexes (Go) and dense bodies (Db). On their luminal surfaces several short microvilli and a single cilium (Cil) are seen. Junctional complexes (Jc) join adjacent cells. Interdigitations occur on the lateral cell surfaces, especially near the base of the cells. In the space between the vein and the bile duct, there are fibrocytes (Fc), collagenous (Cf) and elastic fibers (Ef), a migrating lymphocyte (Mc) and non-myelinated nerve fibers (Nf) enclosed by a Schwann cell.

Bl : Basal lamina.
Dlu : Lumen of bile duct.
R : Erythrocyte.
Vlu : Lumen of interlobular vein.

Liver of a 39-year-old female with cholelithiasis. Obtained by surgical operation. Fixation in 2.0% glutaraldehyde followed by 2.0% osmium tetroxide in phosphate buffer. Uranyl acetate and lead tartarate staining. ×5,000.

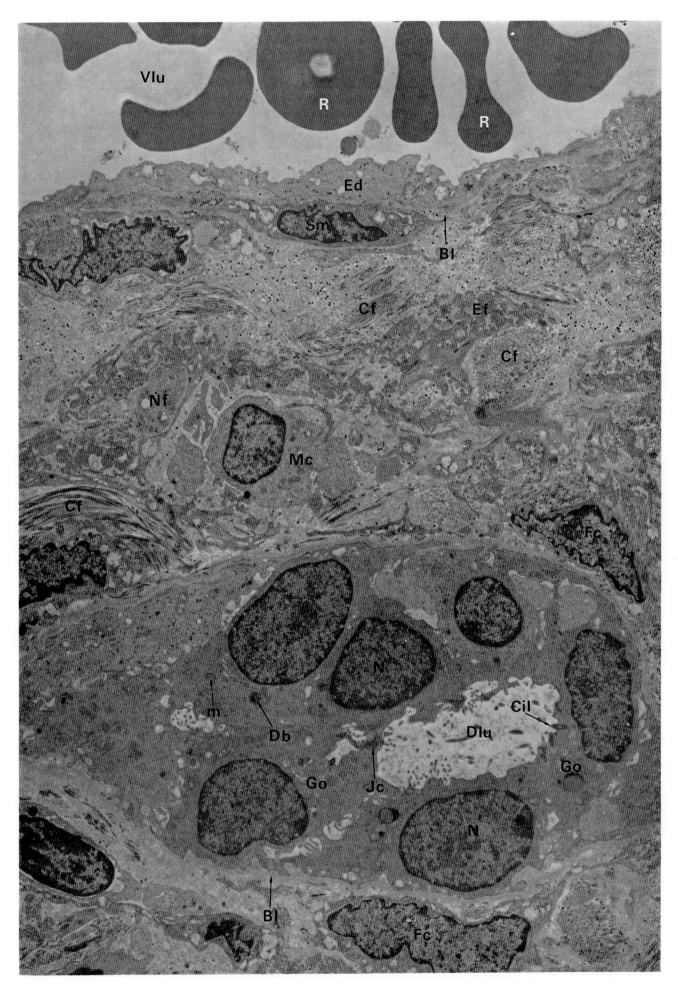

143

Epithelium of the gall bladder

The bile secreted from the liver is stored in the gall bladder, when the sphincter of Oddi is closed between meals, and is considerably concentrated by the reabsorption of water through the epithelium.

The epithelium is composed of simple tall columnar cells provided with many microvilli (Mv) on the luminal surface. The nucleus (N) lies near the cell base. Golgi complexes (Go) occur in the supranuclear region. Mitochondria (m) and free ribosomes are scattered throughout the cytoplasm. Many large dense bodies (Db) are contained in the supranuclear area and also extend to the apical cytoplasm. The adjacent cells are closely joined to one another by a junctional complex (Jc) near the luminal surface. Below this, the lateral cell surfaces possess extensively-pleated foldings (Fo) which partly exhibit elaborated interdigitations. The intercellular space is more or less dilated near the cell base. It has been suggested that the absorption of water and ions from the bile takes place by an active transport process across the lateral cell membrane into the intercellular space. A thin basal lamina (Bl) runs beneath the epithelium.

Cf: Collagenous fiber.
Lu: Lumen.

Surgically-obtained gall bladder of a 39-year-old female with cholelithiasis (silent stone). Phosphate-buffered 2.0% glutaraldehyde fixation followed by 2.0% osmium tetroxide post-fixation. Uranyl acetate and lead tartarate staining. ×6,500.

REFERENCE:

CHAPMAN, G. B., A. J. CHIARODO, R. J. COFFEY and K. WIENEKE: The fine structure of mucosal epithelial cells of a pathological human gall bladder. Anat. Rec., *154*: 579-616, 1966.

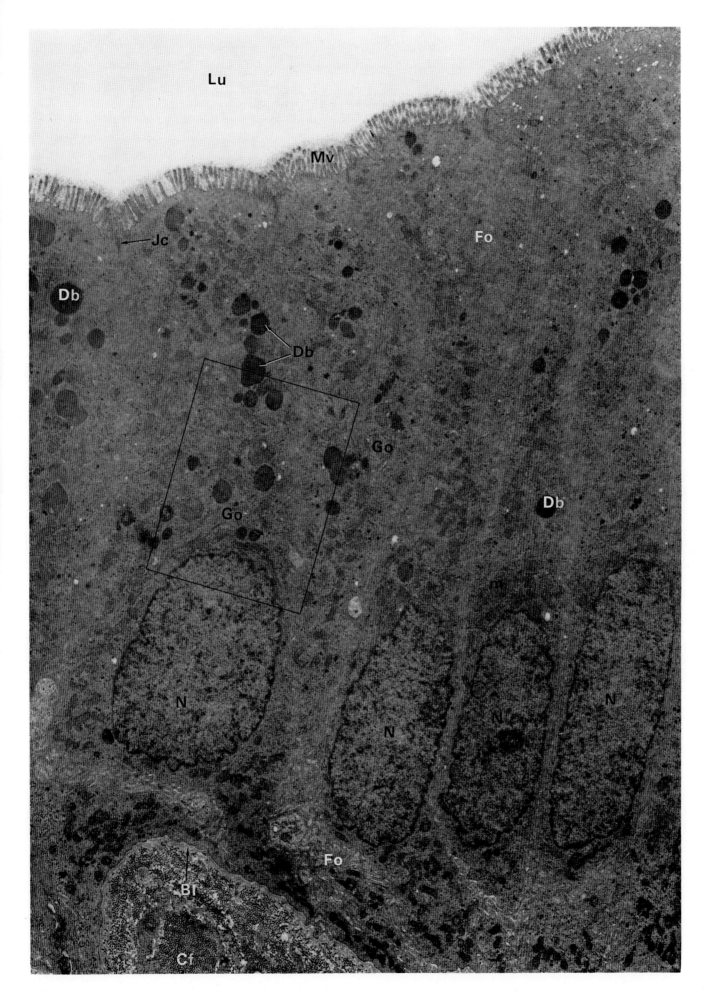

145

Supranuclear portion of the gall bladder epithelial cell

This micrograph is a higher magnification of the area enclosed by a rectangle in the previous picture. The dense bodies (Db) are limited by a single membrane and consist of an accumulation of numerous fine granules. The granular endoplasmic reticulum (Er) is relatively well developed. Within the sacs of Golgi complexes (Go), fine granules similar to the content of the dense bodies are packed (arrow), suggesting an intimate relationship between the Golgi complex and the dense bodies. The cytoplasmic foldings (Fo) of the lateral cell surfaces are partly interdigitated (Id).

      m: Mitochondrion.

      N: Nucleus

Material and method are the same as those of the picture on page 145. ×28,000.

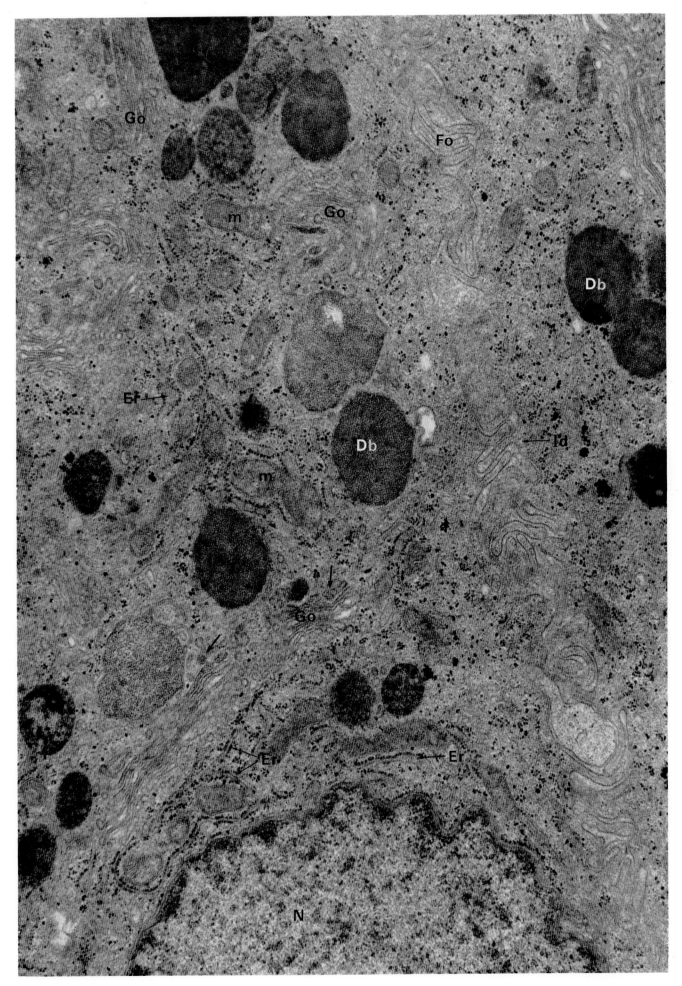

PANCREAS

The pancreas consists of two parts, exocrine and endocrine. The exocrine part is a typical compound acinar gland which secretes the pancreatic juice containing digestive enzymes such as amylase, lipase and trypsin. The endocrine part is the islets of Langerhans that constitute only about one per cent of the total parenchyme of the human pancreas. The endocrine part secretes hormones such as insulin and glucagon.

Interlobular duct of the exocrine pancreas (Top)

The lining of the interlobular duct is composed of a simple low columnar epithelium covered by a thick fibro-connective tissue. The cell contains few organelles in its cytoplasm and bears a few microvilli on the luminal surface.

Bl : Basal lamina.
Cap : Blood capillary.
Cf : Collagenous fiber.

Intercalated duct of the pancreas (Bottom)

The intercalated duct is a thin duct attached to the acinus. Its epithelial cells, like those of the excretory duct, have some microvilli and only a few inconspicuous cell organelles. In this micrograph the basal surface of the epithelium is covered by thin connective tissue on the bottom and left sides and it applies to the exocrine cells on the opposite side. The lumen is filled with a dark secretion of the acinus.

Ac : Acinar cell.
Ld : Lipid droplet.
Lu : Lumen of the intercalated duct.
N : Nucleus.
∗ : Connective tissue.

Top and Bottom : Pancreas of a 59-year-old male with gastric cancer which was obtained by surgical operation. Phosphate-buffered 2.5% glutaraldehyde fixation followed by 1.0% osmium tetroxide post-fixation. Uranyl acetate and lead tartarate staining. Top : ×3,700. Bottom : ×7,000.

REFERENCE :

EKHOLM, R. and Y. EDLUND : Ultrastructure of the human endocrine pancreas. J. Ultrastr. Res., *2* : 453–481, 1959.

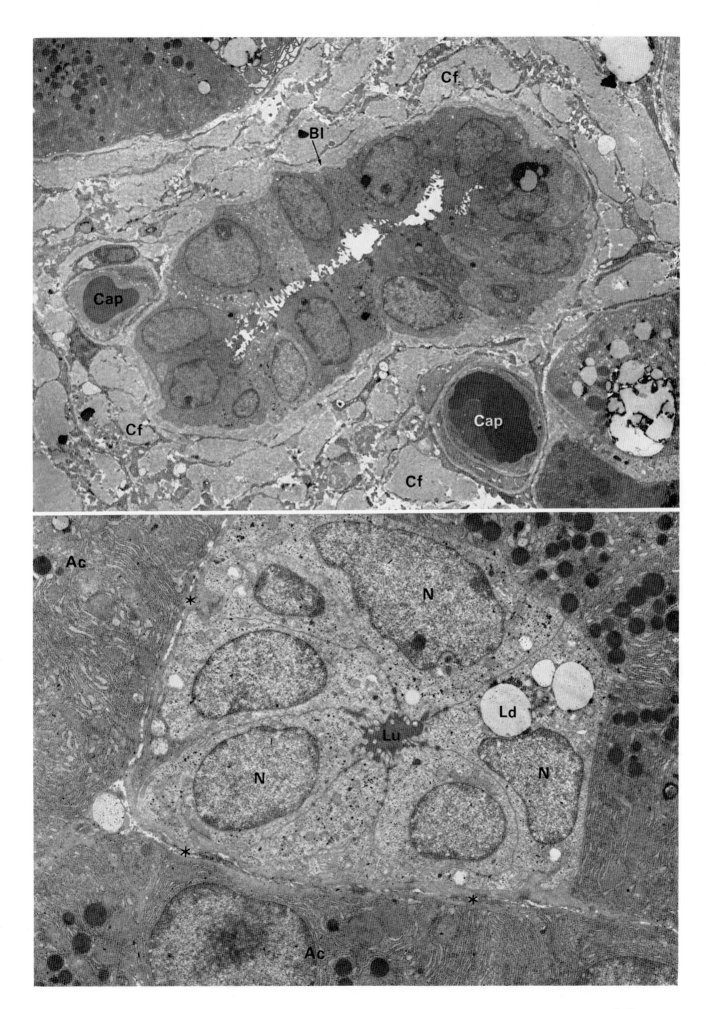

Relation of acinar to centroacinar cell

The pancreatic acini do not become directly continuous with the intercalated ducts, but they tend to surround the beginnings of the ducts on all sides. The duct cells thus taken up into the acini are called centroacinar cells. They have a small, oval nucleus and contain in their cytoplasm a small number of mitochondria, poorly-developed Golgi complexes and a few profiles of granular endoplasmic reticulum. Their cytoplasm generally appears distinctively lighter than that of the acinar cells which have dark secretory granules and abundant granular endoplasmic reticulum.

Top : In this picture are shown two acini drained by an intercalated duct (Icd). The glandular lumen (Glu) is filled with a dark homogeneous secretion. The centroacinar cells (Cac) are continuous to the epithelial cells of the intercalated duct and no clear criterion is found to distinguish them.

Cap : Capillary.

Bottom : A closer view of the acinar (Ac) and centroacinar cells (Cac). A part of the cell surface of the latter faces a basal lamina (Bl). The centroacinar cells in this micrograph contain fairly numerous mitochondria (m) and a small Golgi complex (Go).

Er : Granular endoplasmic reticulum.
Glu : Glandular lumen.
Ly : Lysosome.
m : Mitochondrion.
Nu : Nucleolus.

Top and Bottom : Pancreas of a 68-year-old female with gastric cancer. Obtained by surgical operation. Method for specimen preparation is the same as that of the pictures on page 149. Top: ×2,800. Bottom: ×7,500.

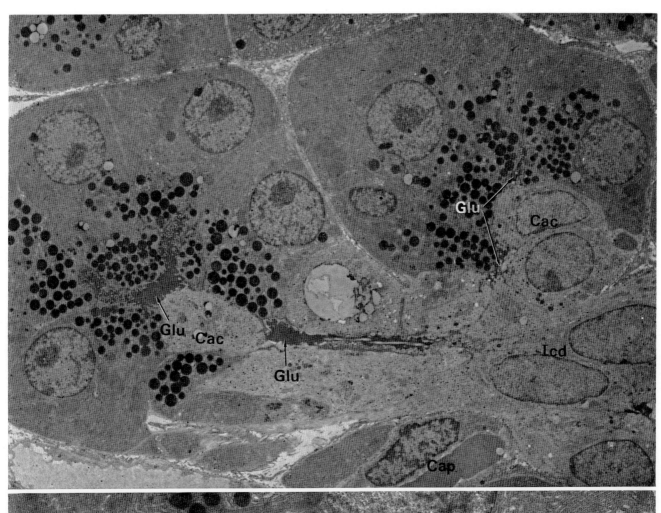

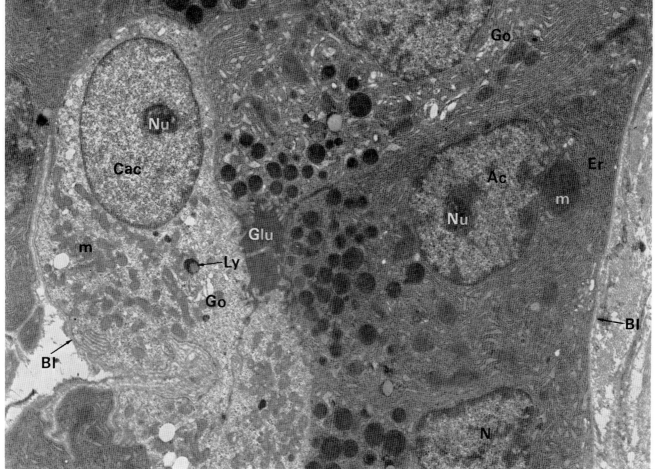

PANCREAS

Acinar cell

The pancreatic acinar cells or exocrine cells are the site of production of the digestive enzymes contained in the pancreatic juice. These cells are roughly pyramidal in shape and constitute the acini or terminal portions of the exocrine part of the pancreas.

The nuclei are central to basal in position and rounded in shape. The nucleoli (Nu) are prominent and large. The apical half of the cells contains a number of rounded, dense, membrane-bounded granules (g). As they contain digestive enzymes, they are called zymogen granules. In the fasting condition, as shown in this picture, the zymogen granules are large in number, but with feeding they are released into the glandular lumen. The basal half of the cells is mostly filled with the granular endoplasmic reticulum (Er) and a few mitochondria (m). Flattened cisterns of granular endoplasmic reticulum are often assembled in parallel arrays. Golgi complexes (Go) consisting of lamellae and vesicles of the smooth-surfaced membrane are located in the supra- and para-nuclear regions. A few lysosomes (Ly) are located between other cell organelles.

In this picture most of the apical surface of the acinar cells is covered by centroacinar cells (Cac) whose cytoplasm contains only a few cell organelles. Several microvilli project into the glandular lumen (Glu) filled with a secretory product of medium density. Junctional complexes (Jc) are located near the luminal surface where adjoining cells meet. The lateral cell surface (*) is smooth, and desmosomes (d) occur here. The base of the cell rests on the basal lamina (Bl).

Material and method are the same as those of the pictures on page 149.   × 13,000.

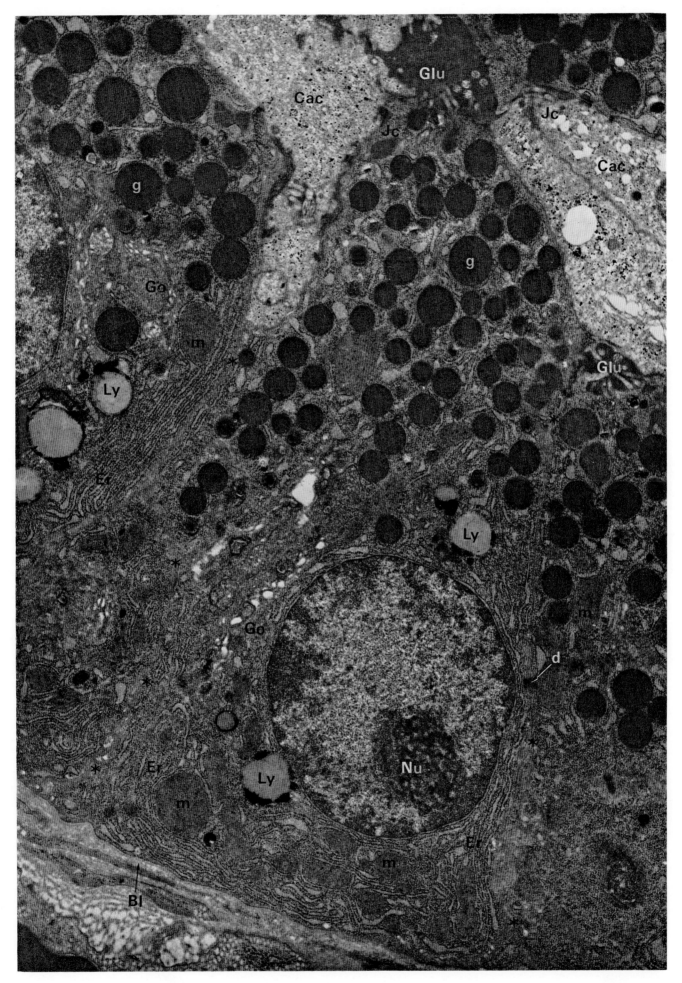

153

Islet of Langerhans

As in other mammals, the human endocrine pancreas consists of three types of secretory cells. The B cells, which are the source of insulin, make up about 70 per cent of the total cell population, whereas the A cells, producing glucagon are about 15 per cent and the D cells, probable source of a third, unidentified hormone, another 15 per cent.

Top: Survey electron micrograph of an islet of Langerhans.

There are two A cells (A) with dense round secretory granules, many B cells (B) containing granules with crystalloid core and two D cells (D) showing large round granules of medium electron density.

Pancreas of a 56-year-old male with cholecystitis. Biopsy material obtained during the cholecystectomy. Phosphate-buffered 2.5% glutaraldehyde fixation followed by post-fixation with 1.3% osmium tetroxide solution. Uranyl acetate and lead tartarate staining. ×4,500.

Bottom: B cell of the islet of Langerhans.

The cell has a round nucleus with a conspicuous nucleolus (Nu). The cytoplasm is filled with numerous specific granules which are believed to contain insulin. The core of the granule is highly pleomorphic and a wide clear space is seen between the core and membrane sac. Occurrence of large lipoidal bodies (Ly) which may be of lysosomal nature is characteristic of the human endocrine pancreas.

Fc: Fibrocyte.
Go: Golgi complex.
m: Mitochondrion.
Nf: Non-myelinated nerve fiber.
Nu: Nucleolus.

Pancreas of a 59-year-old male with gastric cancer. Method for specimen preparation is the same as that of the top picture. ×7,500.

REFERENCES:

GREIDER, M. H., S. A. BENCOSME and J. LECHAGO: The human pancreatic islet cells and their tumors. I. The normal pancreatic islets. Lab. Invest., *22*: 344–354, 1970.

KAWANISHI, H., Y. AKAZAWA and B. MACHI: Islets of Langerhans in normal and diabetic humans. Ultrastructure and histochemistry, with special reference to hyalinosis. Acta pathol jap., *16*: 177–197, 1966.

LIKE, A. A.: The ultrastructure of the secretory cells of the islets of Langerhans in man. Lab. Invest., *16*: 937–951, 1967.

SHIBASAKI, S. and T. ITO: Electron microscopic study on the human pancreatic islets. Arch. histol. jap. *31*: 119–154, 1969.

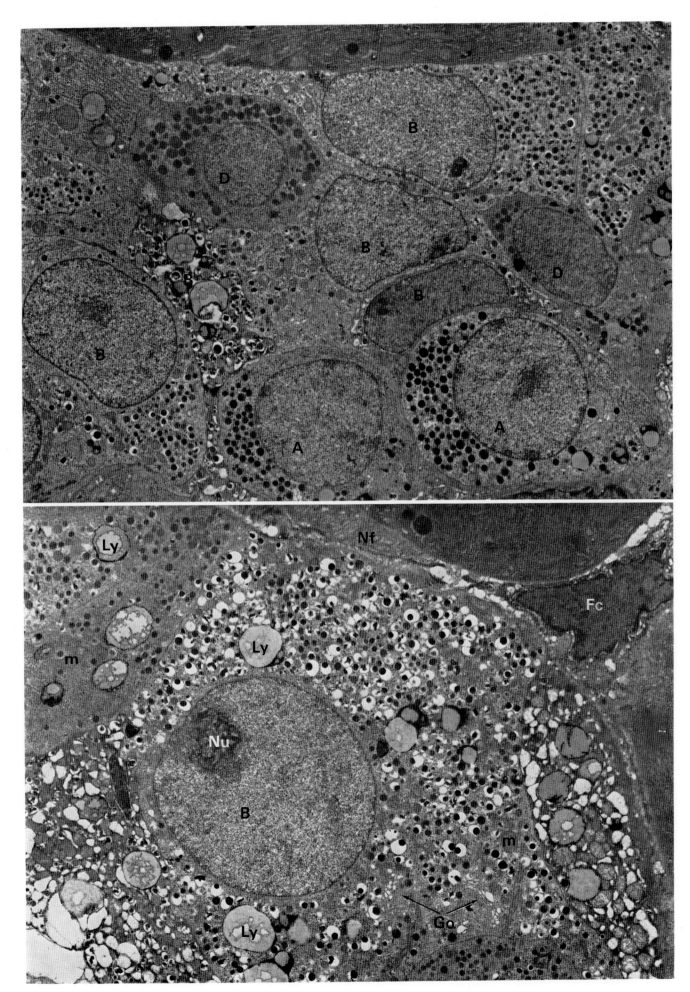

155

Top : A cell of the islet of Langerhans.

Dense round granules, which contain glucagon, are accumulated toward the side of the connective tissue (∗). The granule content consists of a dark round core and a grey substance surrounding it. The significance of this double construction of granules is not yet elucidated. On the opposite side of the cell are flattened sacs of granular endoplasmic reticulum (Er). A considerable number of round mitochondria (m) are scattered among secretory granules. The human A cell is characterized by conspicuous lipoidal bodies, presumably of lysosomal nature (Ly).

Cap : Capillary.
Nu : Nucleolus.

Bottom : D cell of the islet of Langerhans.

The D cell is believed to be a third endocrine element of the pancreatic islet, though its hormone is still unknown. The specific granules are round and moderately electron dense. The double structure in the A cell granules does not occur in this cell type.

In this micrograph the specific granules are gathered on one side of the cell facing the connective tissue space containing a blood capillary (Cap), whereas Golgi complexes (Go), mitochondria (m) and flattened sacs of granular endoplasmic reticulum (Er) are seen on the opposite side. Several large lipoidal bodies (Ly) are seen in the upper portion of this micrograph.

c : Centriole.
Go : Golgi complex.
Nu : Nucleolus.

Top and Bottom : Material and method are the same as those of the top picture on page 155. Top: ×14,000. Bottom : ×10,500.

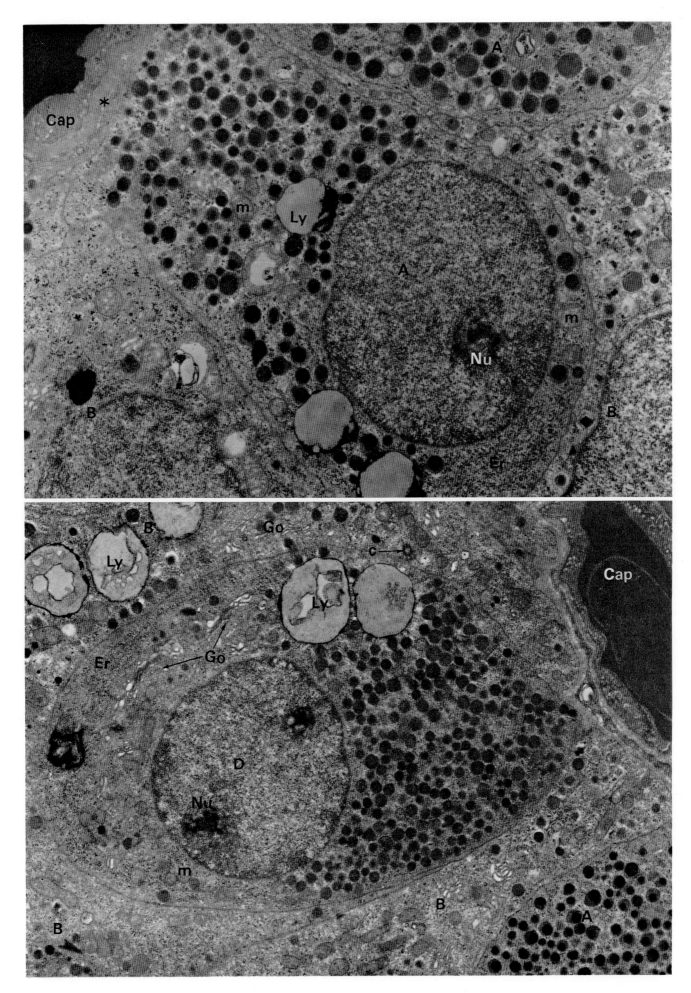

Ciliated cells in the intrapulmonary bronchus

The bronchial epithelium is of a pseudostratified columnar type. It contains ciliated cells, goblet cells, brush cells and basal cells. Among them only basal cells do not reach the lumen. In this electron micrograph apical portions of three ciliated cells are shown. Their free surface is provided with numerous microvilli (Mv), in which much longer and thicker cilia are mingled. The latter are originated from the basal bodies (Bb) accompanied by rootlets (Rt). Mitochondria (m) are numerous in the apical cytoplasm. Dense bodies (Db) are present in the supranuclear region.

Cil : Cilium.
d : Desmosome.
Er : Granular endoplasmic reticulum.
Jc : Junctional complex.
N : Nucleus of the ciliated cell.

Surgically-obtained intrapulmonary bronchus of a 72-year-old male with bronchial cancer. Fixation in phosphate-buffered 2.5% glutaraldehyde followed by 2.0% osmium tetroxide post-fixation. Uranyl acetate and lead citrate staining. ×15,000. (Photograph courtesy of Dr. H. Ozawa)

REFERENCE:

Frasca, J. M., O. Auerbach, V. R. Parks, and W. Stoeckenius: Electron microscopic observations of bronchial epithelium. 1. Annulate lamellae. Exp. molec. Pathol., 6: 261–273, 1967.

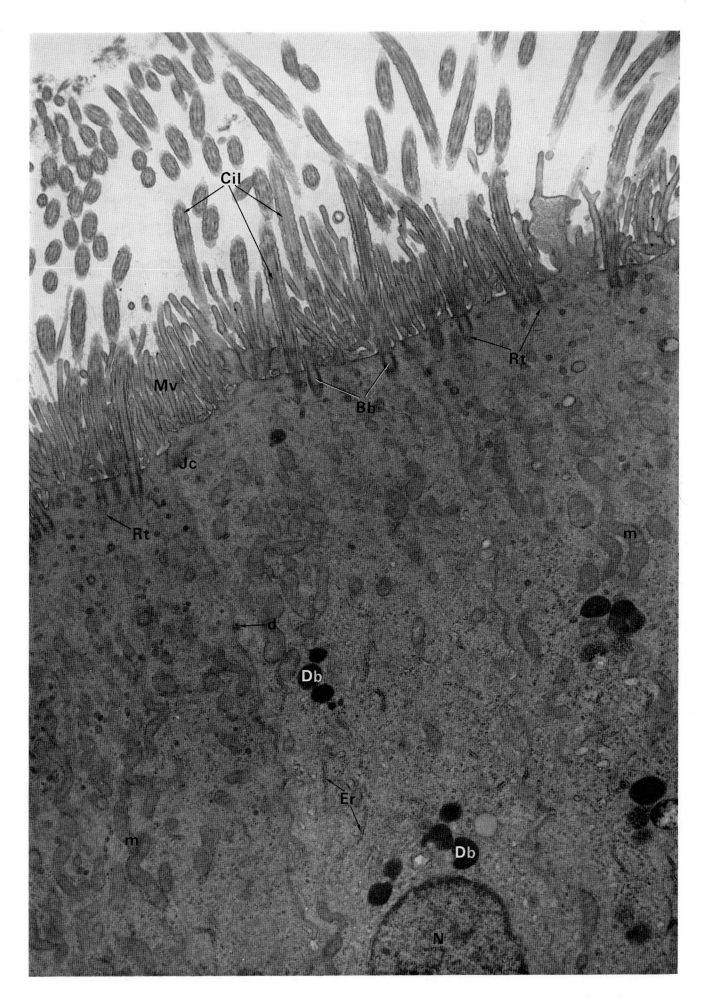

159

Cilia

As is the rule throughout the animal kingdom, the human cilium contains two central fibrils and nine pairs of peripheral fibrils. The fibrils, which appear tubular in cross section, are the continuation of the basal bodies in the apical cytoplasm. The beating movement of the cilia is believed to be caused by the contraction of rootlets which are obliquely attached to the basal bodies.

Top: Cross section through the cilia in the bronchiolar epithelium. The regular 9+1 pattern of cilia fibrils is clearly seen.

Cf: Central fibril.
Pf: Peripheral fibril.

Lung of a 26-year-old male with mediastinal tumor. This material was obtained by surgical operation. Fixation in 2.0% glutaraldehyde followed by post-fixation with 2.0% osmium tetroxide in cacodylate buffer. Uranyl acetate and lead tartarate staining. ×72,000.

Bottom: Longitudinal section through the apex of ciliated cells of the bronchial epithelium. In this micrograph three cilia (Cil) and numerous microvilli (Mv) are shown. The fibrils, which are originated from the basal body (Bb), run to the tip of the cilium. The rootlet (Rt), which is striated, extends from the basal body into the apical cytoplasm. The microvilli divide into branches like cactus.

Zo: Zonula occludens of a junctional complex

Material and method are the same as those of the picture on page 159. ×68,000. (Photograph courtesy of Dr. H. Ozawa)

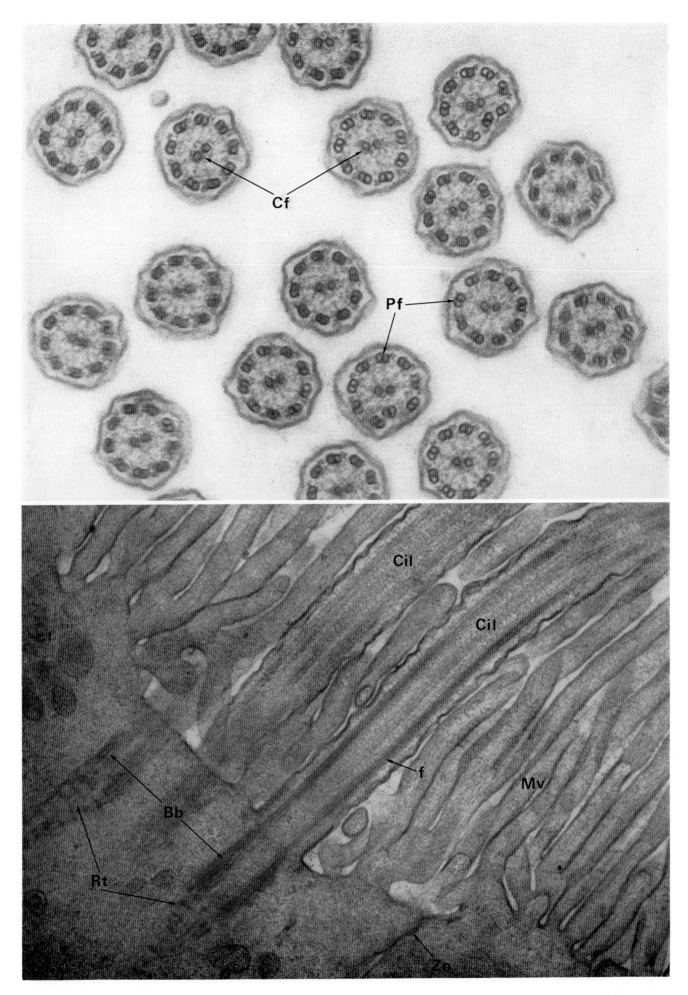

Bronchial gland

The surface of the bronchus is moistened by the secretion of the bronchial glands. These are small, mixed type glands usually located beneath the muscular layer of the bronchus.

Top: This micrograph shows glandular cells of a serous type. The nucleus (N) is located basally. Secretory granules (Sg) are accumulated in the apical cytoplasm. They vary in size and electron density. Large Golgi complexes (Go) are located in the supranuclear region, and conspicuous granular endoplasmic reticulum (Er) occurs around the nucleus. The lateral cell membranes possess small cytoplasmic processes. A basal lamina (Bl) covers the outside of the epithelium.

Glu: Glandular lumen.
m: Mitochondrion.

Bottom: A basal portion of a mucous cell and a myoepithelial cell of the bronchial gland. The mucous secretory granules (Mg), which are less dense than the serous ones shown in the upper micrograph, occupy most of the cytoplasm so that the nucleus (Ne) is pushed basally. Granular endoplasmic reticulum (Er) and a Golgi complex (Go) occur within the narrowed cytoplasm between the granules.

The myoepithelial cell is situated between the mucous cell and the basal lamina (Bl). Its cell body and nucleus (Nm) are elongate in shape. The cytoplasm is largely occupied by fine filaments (f) which represent the contractile element of this cell and are usually oriented in large bundles extended longitudinally. In the cytoplasm near the basal lamina, numerous small vesicles occur. Desmosomes (d) are formed between the mucous and myoepithelial cells.

Top and Bottom: Bronchus surgically obtained from a 72-year-old male with bronchial cancer. Fixation in 2.0% glutaraldehyde followed by post-fixation in 2.0% osmium tetroxide in phosphate buffer. Uranyl acetate and lead tartarate staining. Top: ×8,500. Bottom: ×10,500.

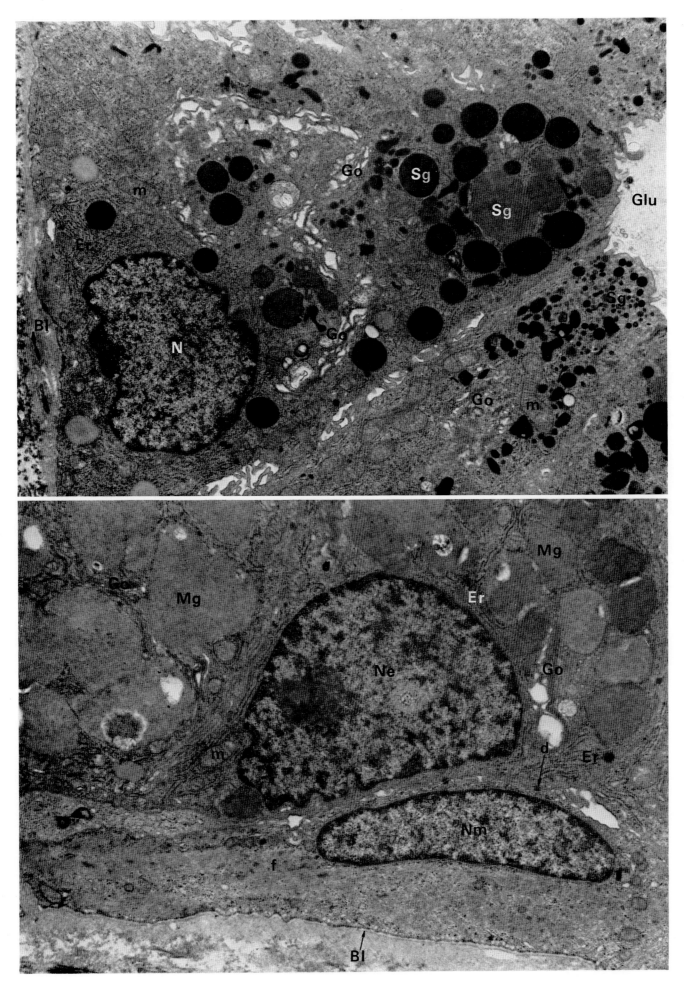

Ciliated cell in the bronchiole

This micrograph shows ciliated cells of the terminal bronchiole. The free surface is provided with many microvilli (Mv) and several cilia (Cil). The nucleus (N) is located near the cell base. Golgi complexes (Go), mitochondria (m) and lysosomes (Ly) are present in the supranuclear region. An accumulation of glycogen particles (Gl) is seen in the supra and infranuclear region.

Blu: Bronchiolar lumen.
Bl: Basal lamina.
Jc: Junctional complex.
Ld: Lipid droplet.

Lung of a 26-year-old male with mediastinal tumor. Obtained by surgical operation. Fixation in 2.0% glutaraldehyde followed by 2.0% osmium tetroxide in cacodylate buffer. Uranyl acetate and lead tartarate staining. ×12,000.

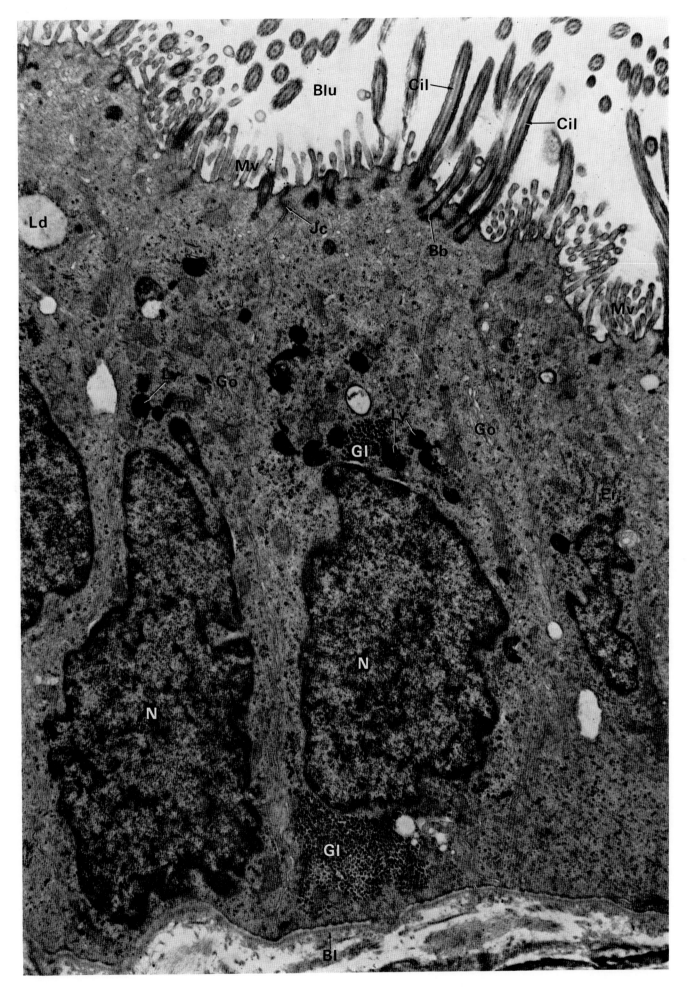

Secretory cell and other cells in the terminal bronchiole (Top)

In the bronchiole the goblet cell, which is an important component of the tracheal and the bronchial epithelia, is supplanted by another type of secretory cell. This type of cell (Sc), which is seen between ciliated cells (Cc) in this micrograph, is low columnar in shape and has an ovoid nucleus (N). A few short microvilli (Mv) occur on the free surface. Apically, the lateral cell membrane is closely attached to the adjacent ciliated cell by a junctional complex (Jc). A number of secretory granules (Sg) with high electron density are accumulated within the apical cytoplasm. Golgi complexes (Go) and granular endoplasmic reticulum (Er) are in the supranuclear region. Figures suggesting the formation of secretory granules in the Golgi area are seen (arrow). A cell possessing round bodies bound in a single membrane (Sb) is seen in the upper left corner of this picture. They contain tangled string-like material.

    Blu: Bronchiolar lumen.
    Bl: Basal lamina.
    m: Mitochondrion.

Epithelium of the respiratory bronchiole (Bottom)

The respiratory bronchiole is lined by cuboidal epithelial cells. In this micrograph three types of cells are recognizable: ciliated, brush and secretory cells. The ciliated cell (Cc) is provided with a few cilia (Cil) and scanty microvilli (Mv) on its free surface. The brush cell (Bc) is covered by numerous microvilli, and contains large dense bodies (Db) of lysosomal nature in the supranuclear region. The secretory cell has a large nucleus and moderately developed granular endoplasmic reticulum. A few secretory granules (Sg) are present apically. Microvilli are relatively sparse on the free surface. The lateral cell membranes of adjacent cells are apically closed with one another by a junctional complex (Jc).

    Blu: Bronchiolar lumen.
    Go: Golgi complex.
    N: Nucleus.

Top and Bottom: Material and method are the same as those of the previous picture. Top: ×6,000. Bottom: ×8,000.

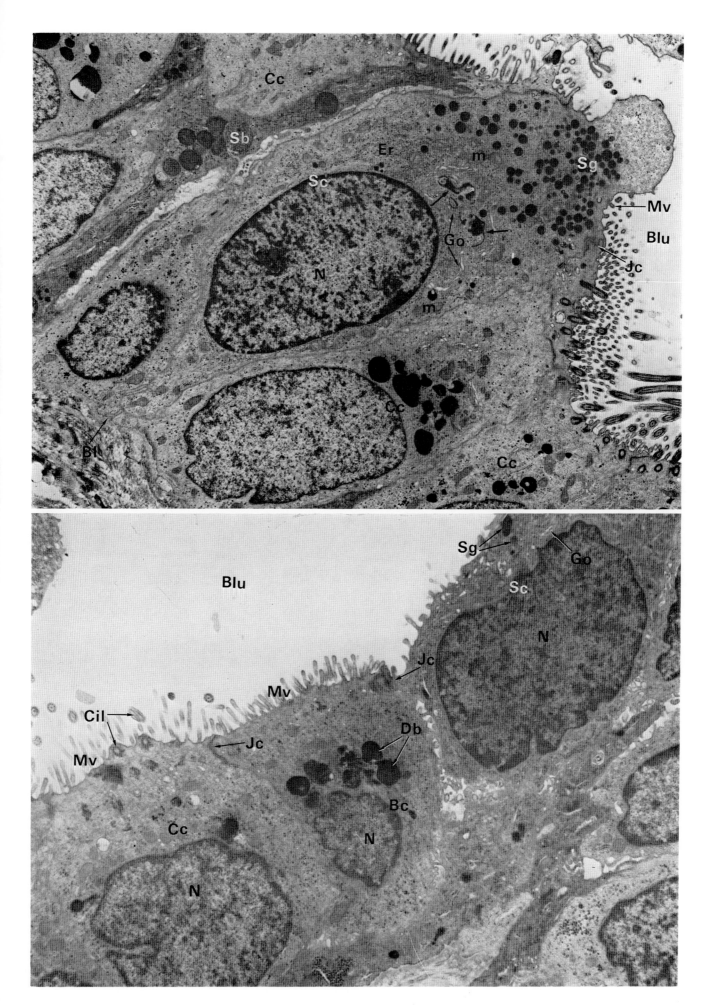

Alveolar duct

The alveolar duct, to which many alveoli open, is an air passage subsequent to the respiratory bronchiole. Smooth muscles extend from the respiratory bronchiole along the duct to end in a sphincter at the terminal portion of the duct.

Top: This micrograph shows a longitudinal section of the alveolar duct wall near the respiratory bronchiole. The wall is composed of smooth muscles (Sm), fibrocytes (Fc), elastic (Ef) and collagenous fibers (Cf). On the left side is seen the duct lumen (Dlu) where the air passes. The lumen of an alveolus (Alu) is shown in the upper right corner. Capillaries (Cap) which are covered by the squamous epithelial cell (Sc) swell into the air spaces.

> Ed: Endothelial cell.
> Gc: Great alveolar cell.
> R: Erythrocyte.

Material and method are the same as those of the picture on page 165. ×4,500.

Bottom: This micrograph shows a cross section of a sphincter of the alveolar duct. It protrudes into the alveolar duct from the tip of an alveolar wall (Aw), and is composed of a bundle of smooth muscles (Sm), elastic fibers (Ef) and collagenous fibers (Cf). A thin cytoplasmic layer of the squamous alveolar epithelial cells (Sc) extends from the alveolar wall to cover the sphincter. A single layer of the basal lamina (Bl) which is also continuous to that of the alveolar wall runs beneath the epithelial layer. The sphincter is presumed to contribute to the prevention of excess expansion of alveolar ducts and sacs, and also to their contraction at the time of expiration.

> Fp: Process of fibrocyte.

Lung of an 11-year-old female with diaphragmatic hernia. Obtained by surgical operation. Fixation in 2.0% osmium tetroxide in s-collidine buffer. Lead tartarate staining. ×6,000.

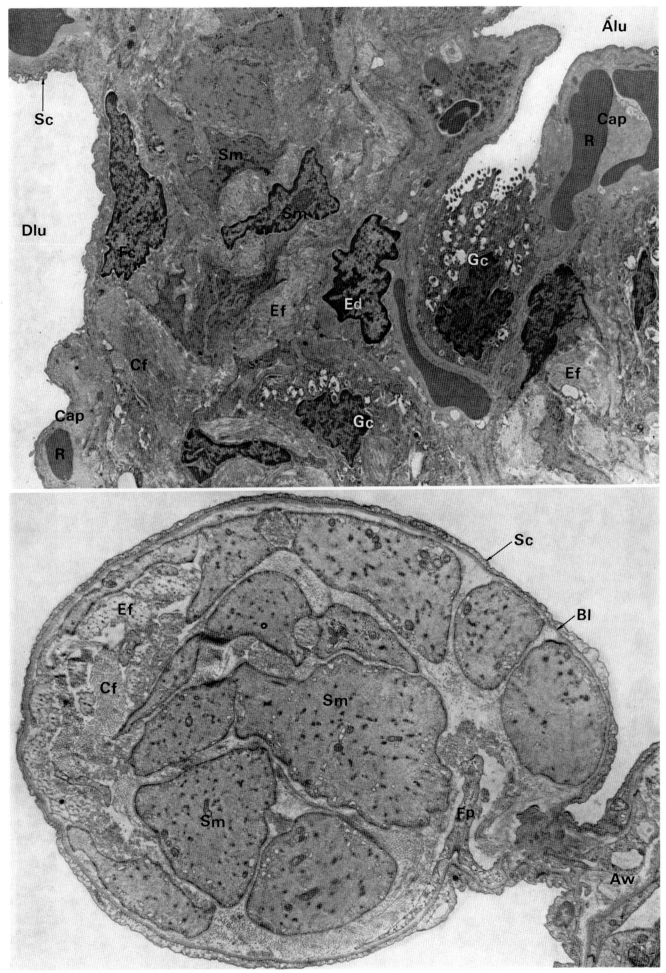

Alveolar wall

The lung has a structural pattern similar to that of a compound alveolar gland. The bronchus and its branches correspond to the duct system, whereas the alveoli are the terminal portion. There are up to 400 million alveoli in the lung, and adjacent alveoli are separated by a thin alveolar wall.

The alveolar wall is composed of an alveolar epithelium, capillaries (Cap), and connective tissue elements. The alveolar epithelium consists of two types of cells: the squamous alveolar epithelial cell (Sc) extending its thin cytoplasmic process over the capillary wall and the great alveolar epithelial cell (Gc) characterized by lamellar bodies (Lb) in the cytoplasm. In the space limited by basal laminae underlying the alveolar epithelium and covering the blood capillaries, there are collagenous fibers (Cf), elastic fibers (Ef) and profiles of connective tissue cells. In many regions, the capillaries are related so closely to squamous alveolar epithelial cells, that their respective basal laminae fuse into one layer called alveolar basement membrane (Abm). Gaseous exchange between the blood and the air is believed to occur through the greatly attenuated cytoplasm of the squamous alveolar epithelial cell, the fused (single) alveolar basement membrane and the attenuated cytoplasm of the capillary endothelial cell.

Alu: Alveolar lumen.
Am: Alveolar membrane (So-called blood-air barrier).
Ed: Endothelial cell.
Fc: Fibrocyte.
R: Erythrocyte.

Material and method are the same as those of the picture on page 165. ×10,000.

REFERENCES:

Campiche, M. A., A. Gautier, E. I. Hernandez and A. Reymond: An electron microscopic study of the fetal development of human lung. Pediatrics, *32*: 976-994, 1963.

Hayek, H.: Die menschliche Lunge. Springer-Verlag, Berlin, 1970.

Low, F. N.: The pulmonary alveolar epithelium of laboratory mammals and man. Anat. Rec., *117*: 241-263, 1953.

Weibel, E. R.: The mystery of "non-nucleated plates" in the alveolar epithelium of the lung explained. Acta anat., *78*: 425-443, 1971.

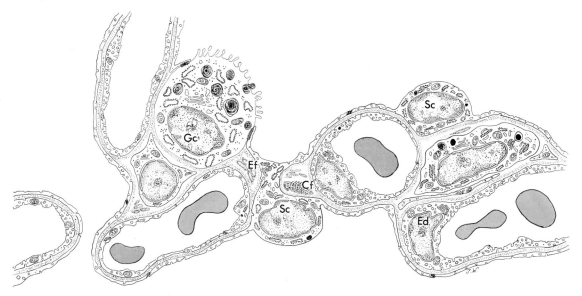

Diagram of the alveolar wall
Cf: Collagenous fiber. Ed: Endothelial cell of the blood capillary. Ef: Elastic fiber.
Gc: Great alveolar epithelial cell. Sc: Squamous alveolar epithelial cell.

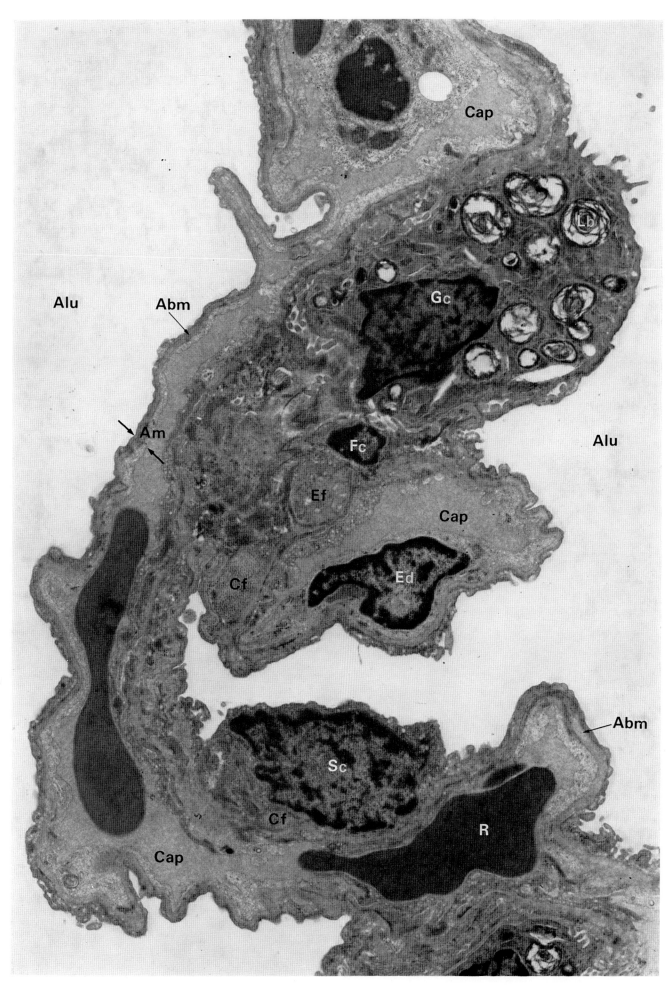

171

Squamous alveolar epithelial cell (Top)

The large ovoid nucleus of the squamous alveolar epithelial cell is covered by a thin cytoplasm with Golgi complexes (Go) and small mitochondria (m) and is located either in the niche portion between capillaries or on the capillary wall. No microvilli can be seen on the free surface of the cell. At the margin of the perinuclear region, the cell is abruptly attenuated into a thin cytoplasmic layer (Asc) covering the alveolar capillaries.

> Alu: Alveolar lumen.
> Bl: Basal lamina.
> Clu: Capillary lumen.
> N: Nucleus.

Material and method are the same as those of the bottom micrograph on page 169. ×19,000.

Alveolar membrane (Middle and Bottom)

The alveolar membrane is also called blood-air barrier as it separates the capillary blood and the alveolar air. Respiratory gases are exchanged between them. This membrane consists of an attenuated cytoplasmic layer of the squamous alveolar epithelial cell (Asc), a thin sheet of the endothelial cell (Ed) and a homogeneous-looking basement membrane (Bm) interposed between them. The endothelium varies in thickness from portion to portion. Where the endothelial cell becomes extremely attenuated, no cell organelles can be found within the cytoplasm, as shown in the middle micrograph. However, in its thicker portions, the cell is provided with numerous vesicles (v) and caveolae (c), as shown in the bottom micrograph.

> Alu: Alveolar lumen.
> R: Erythrocyte.

Material and method are the same as those of the picture on page 165. Middle and Bottom: ×36,000.

REFERENCES:

GRONIOWSKI, J. and W. BICZYSKOWA: Ultrastructure of the blood-air barrier of the neonatal human lungs. Electron microscopy. Proc. 5th Internat. Congr. Electron Microscopy. Philadelphia, 1962, Vol. 2. New York, Academic Press, 1962. pp. WW-5

LOW, F. N.: The extracellular portion of the human blood-air barrier and its relation to tissue space. Anat. Rec., *139*: 105-123, 1961.

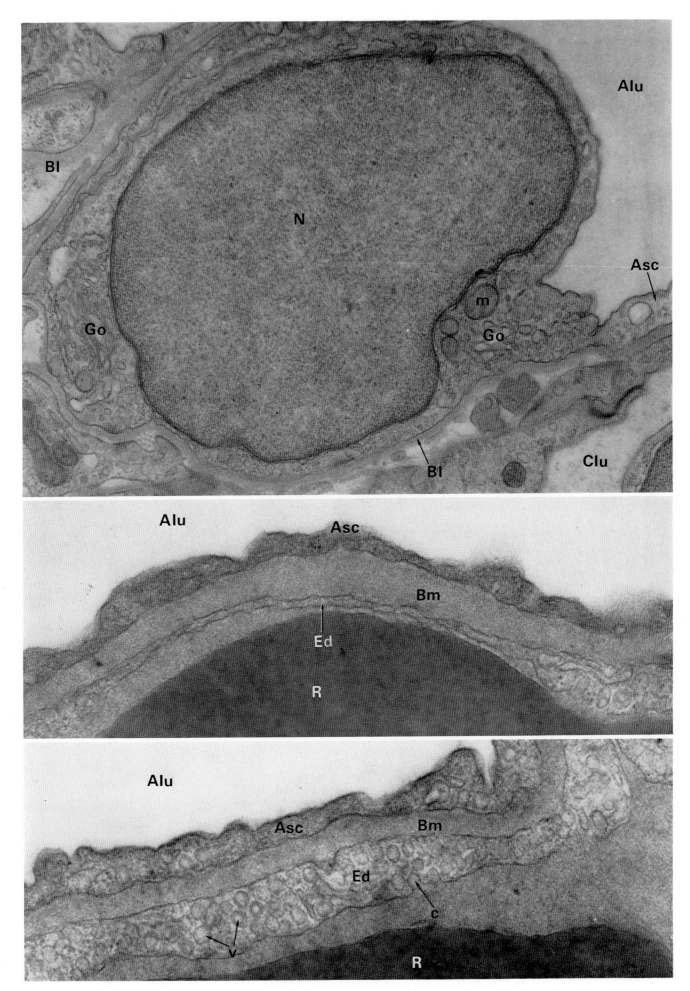

Great alveolar epithelial cell

Top: The great alveolar epithelial cell is usually situated in the alveolar niche between capillaries. This cell is roughly cuboidal in shape and provided with irregular short microvilli (Mv) on its free surface. The most striking feature of this cell is the presence of numerous lamellar bodies (Lb) which are a kind of secretory granule and are thought to contain alveolar surfactant. This cell is tightly attached to the adjacent squamous epithelial cell (Sc) by a junctional complex (Jc). It rests on the basal lamina (Bl) that is continuous with the basement membrane of the alveolar membrane.

Alu: Alveolar lumen.
Clu: Capillary lumen.
Go: Golgi complex.
Hc: Histiocyte.
m: Mitochondrion.
N: Nucleus.

Material and method are the same as those of the bottom micrograph on page 169. ×9,500.

Bottom left: A basal portion of a great alveolar cell. The cytoplasm contains granular endoplasmic reticulum (Er), Golgi complexes (Go) and numerous free ribosomes. Several multivesicular bodies (Mvb), which are thought to be precursors of lamellar bodies (Lb), are present.

Bl: Basal lamina.
m: Mitochondrion.
Nu: Nucleolus.

Material and method are the same as those of the bottom micrograph on page 169. ×18,000.

Bottom right: An apical portion of a great alveolar cell. Here, one may see how the sac of the lamellar body (Lb) opens to the alveolar surface to release its content.

Alu: Alveolar lumen.
m: Mitochondrion.
Mv: Microvillus.
N: Nucleus.

Lung of a 43-year-old female with rheumatoid lung disease. Obtained by open lung biopsy for diagnostic purpose. Fixation in 2.0% glutaraldehyde followed by 2.0% osmium tetroxide in cacodylate buffer. Lead tartarate staining. ×14,000.

REFERENCES:

BALIS, J. U. and P. E. CONEN: The role of alveolar inclusion bodies in the developing lung. Lab. Invest., *13*: 1215–1229, 1964.

BOMMER, W.: Studies on the "laminated bodies" in the alveolar epithelium of human lung. Ann. Paediat. (Basel), *199*: 502–513, 1962.

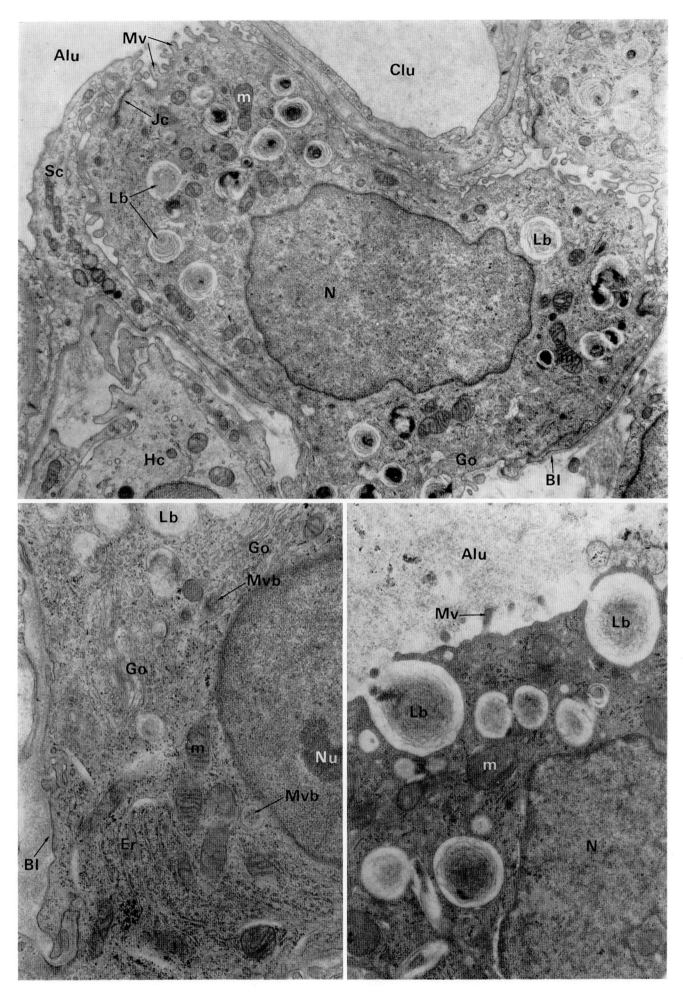

Alveolar macrophage

An alveolar macrophage occurs as a free cell within the alveolar lumen. It is usually mononuclear and characterized by the ability to phagocytize bacteria, minute dusts and other particulate foreign matters, as well as cellular debris. The macrophage containing numerous phagocytized dust particles is called dust cell, whereas that containing large amount of hemosiderin, an iron containing substance resulting from ingested erythrocytes in the case of cardiac insufficiency, is called heart failure cell. Generally speaking, macrophages increase in number when inflammation occurs in the lung.

Top: Common type of the alveolar macrophage. The nucleus (N) is spherical in shape with some indentation. Several cytoplasmic processes (p) are seen around the cytoplasm. It is characteristic of the macrophage that within the cytoplasm there are numerous lysosomes (Ly) of various sizes. These lysosomes are limited by a single membrane and contain internal dense granules. Occasionally the content of the lysosomes reveals a myelin figure (Mf). Mitochondria (m) are small in size and usually scattered around the nucleus. Numerous vesicles (v) are present within the peripheral cytoplasm.

> Alu: Alveolar lumen.
> Aw: Alveolar wall.

Material and method are the same as those of the bottom micrograph on page 169. ×9,000.

Bottom: Stimulated type of the alveolar macrophage. The nucleus is irregular in shape. The long cytoplasmic processes (p) projected from the peripheral cytoplasm are increased in number. Small mitochondria (m) are numerous and the elements of granular endoplasmic reticulum (Er) are well developed. The characteristic lysosomes (Ly) are rather small in diameter, extremely abundant, and have a tendency to gather on one side of the cytoplasm. Golgi complexes (Go) are located in the indented portion of the nucleus. Numerous tonofilaments (f) are seen in the cytoplasm.

> Alu: Alveolar lumen.

Lung of a 57-year-old male with pulmonary fibrosis. Obtained by an open lung biopsy for diagnostic purpose. Fixation with 2.0% glutaraldehyde followed by 2.0% osmium tetroxide in cacodylate buffer. Lead tartarate staining. ×9,000.

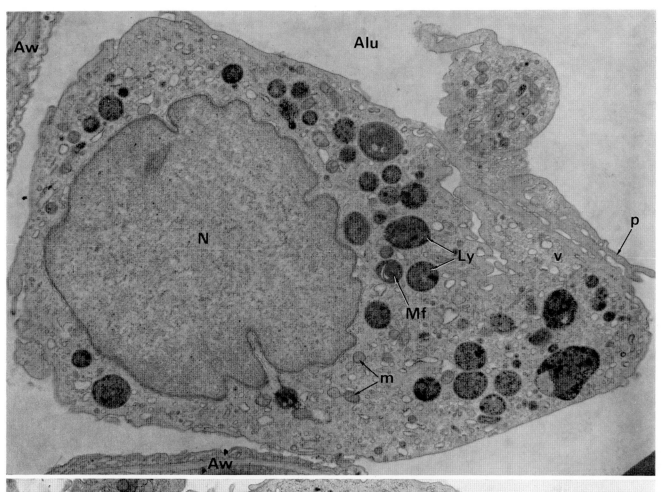

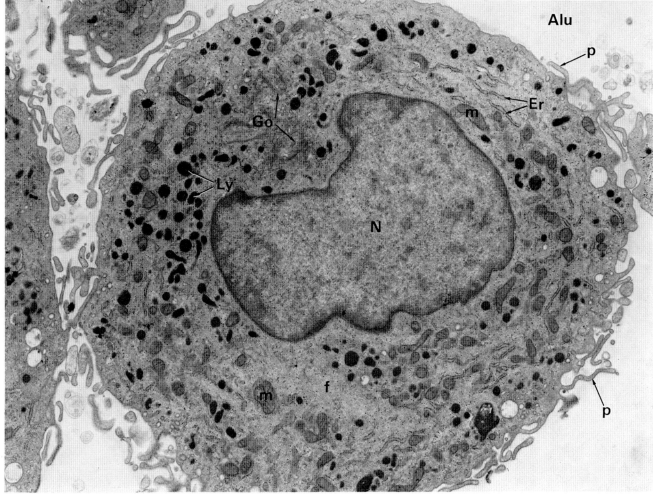

177

KIDNEY

Renal glomerulus

The glomerulus is the portion of the kidney where urine production begins. From the glomerular capillaries a fluid called glomerular filtrate comes into the space of Bowman's capsule. This filtrate changes in its contents during the passage through the subsequent tubules to become urine.

Cell components constituting the glomerulus are capillary endothelial cells (Ed), glomerular epithelial cells (Ep) and mesangial cells (Mes). A single-layered and continuous basement membrane (Bm) is interposed between the endothelial cells and the epithelial cells, and also between the latter and the mesangial cells. The urinary space (Us) lies outside the glomerular epithelia.

Clu: Capillary lumen.

Kidney of a 27-year-old female with movable kidney. Obtained by surgical operation. Fixation with 2.0% osmium tetroxide in s-collidine buffer. Lead tartarate staining. ×4,500.

REFERENCES:

BERGSTRAND, A. and H. BUCHT: Anatomy of the glomerulus observed in biopsy material from young and healthy human subjects. Z. Zellforsch., *48*: 51-73, 1958.

FUJISAKI, S.: Electron microscopic study of glomerulus. Jap. J. Nephrol., *3*: 351-382, 1961. (in Japanese)

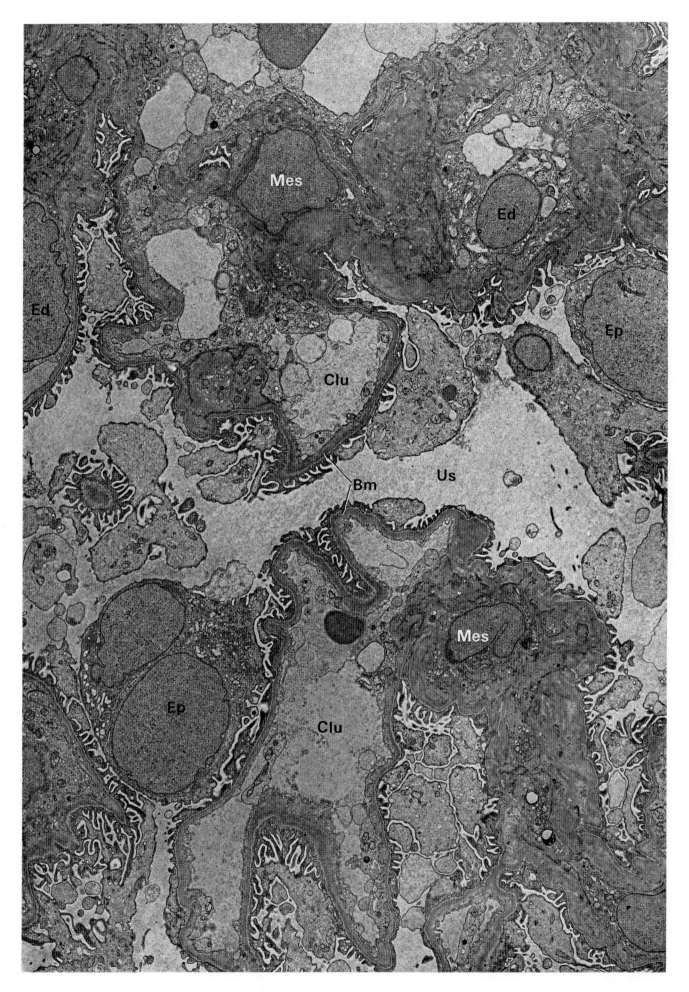

179

Relationship between the mesangium and the glomerular capillaries

The mesangium is a complex of mesangial cells (Mes) and intercellular matrix (Mat). It functions as the supporting element of the glomerular capillaries. Only the nuclear portion of the endothelial cells (Ed) extrudes into the capillary lumen. Their attenuated cytoplasmic sheet lining the capillary lumen is fenestrated. The foot processes (Fp) of the glomerular epithelial cells (Ep) cover the capillary walls and the free parts of the mesangium.

Bm : Basement membrane.
Clu : Capillary lumen.
N : Nucleus.
Us : Urinary space.

Kidney of a 24-year-old female with movable kidney. Obtained by a surgical operation. Fixation with 2.0% osmium tetroxide in s-collidine buffer. Lead tartarate staining. ×11,000.

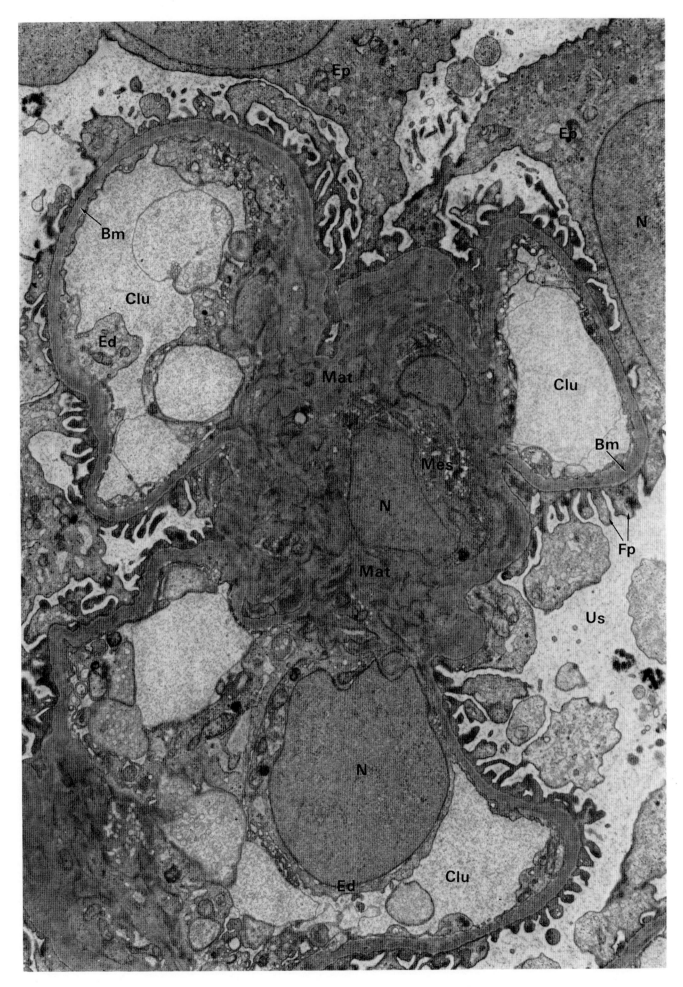

181

Mesangium

The mesangial cell is irregular in shape, exhibiting radiating cytoplasmic processes. As shown in this micrograph, a cell having two nuclei (N) is sometimes found in a plane of a section. The cell has well-developed granular endoplasmic reticulum (Er). Round- or rod-shaped mitochondria (m) are gathered around the nucleus. Vesicles (v) occur abundantly in the peripheral cytoplasm. Numerous fine tonofilaments (f) are contained in the peripheral processes of the cell. Paired centrioles (c) are seen near the nuclei. Several dense bodies (Db), probably of lysosomal nature, are present. The intercellular mesangial matrix (Mat) is continuous with the basement membrane (Bm) and shows fine fibrous structure.

> Ed: Endothelial cell.
> Ep: Epithelial cell.
> Us: Urinary space.

Material and method are the same as those of the picture on page 179.　×16,000.

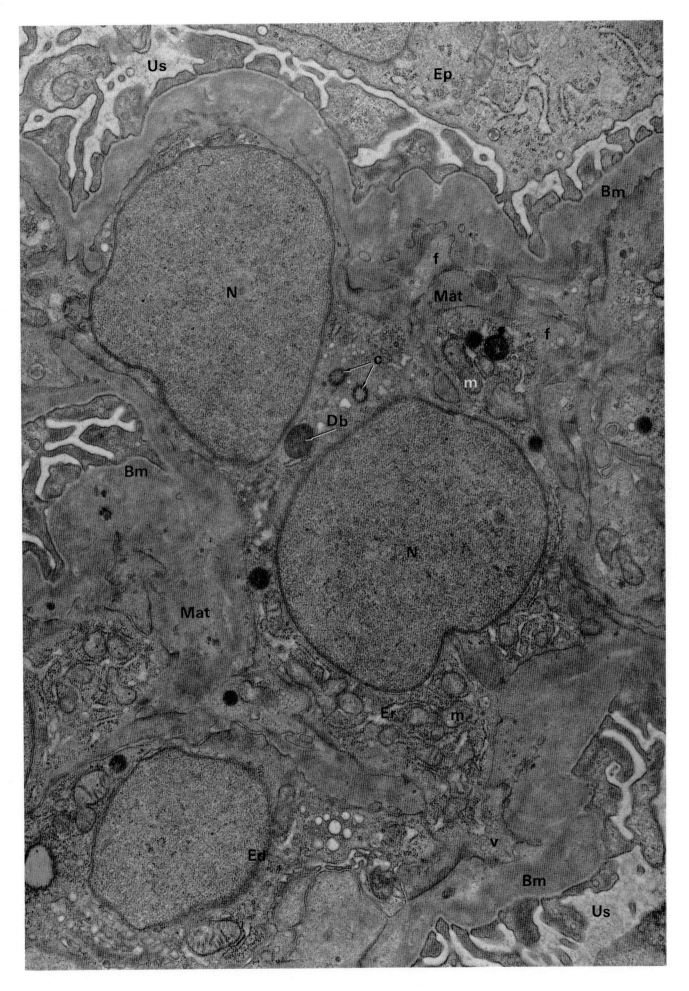

Glomerular epithelial cell (**podocyte**) (Top)

Glomerular epithelial cells cover the glomerular capillaries and the mesangial regions. The perikaryon of the cell is largely occupied by the nucleus (N) with a prominent nucleolus (Nu). Mitochondria (m) are scattered around the nucleus. The perikaryon issues thick cytoplasmic processes from which numerous foot processes (Fp) emerge to attach to the basement membrane (Bm). Occasionally the foot processes originate directly from the perikaryon to end on the capillary wall. Each foot process is separated from the others by a narrow slit (arrow).

Clu : Capillary lumen.
Ed : Endothelial cell.
Ly : Lysosome.
Us : Urinary space.

Material and method are the same as those of the picture on page 179.　×12,000.

Glomerular filtration membrane (Bottom)

The glomerular filtration membrane consists of the epithelial foot processes (Fp), the attenuated cytoplasmic layer of the endothelial cell (Ed) and the basement membrane (Bm) interposing between them.

The so-called basement membrane of the glomerular capillary wall is composed of three layers: electron lucent thin layers immediately beneath the epithelial and endothelial cells and a thick, electron dense layer called lamina densa sandwiched between them.

The slits between the foot processes of the epithelial cell are closed by a thin diaphragm called slit membrane (Sm). The attenuated cytoplasmic thin sheet of the endothelial cells is numerously fenestrated. The endothelial fenestrations are also closed by a thin diaphragm (Di), though it can be seen clearly only in a few places in this micrograph. The final urine-dialyzing membrane is generally believed to consist of the basement membrane and the diaphragms closing the endothelial fenestrations and the slits between the foot processes.

Ep : Epithelial cell.
R : Erythrocyte.
Us : Urinary space.

Material and fixation are the same as those of the picture on page 179. Uranyl acetate and lead tartarate staining.　×27,000.

REFERENCES :

Jørgensen, F.: Electron microscopic studies of normal visceral epithelial cells. Lab. Invest., *17:* 225–242, 1967.

Jørgensen, F. and M. W. Bentzon: The ultrastructure of the normal human glomerulus: Thickness of glomerular basement membrane. Lab. Invest., *18:* 42–48, 1968.

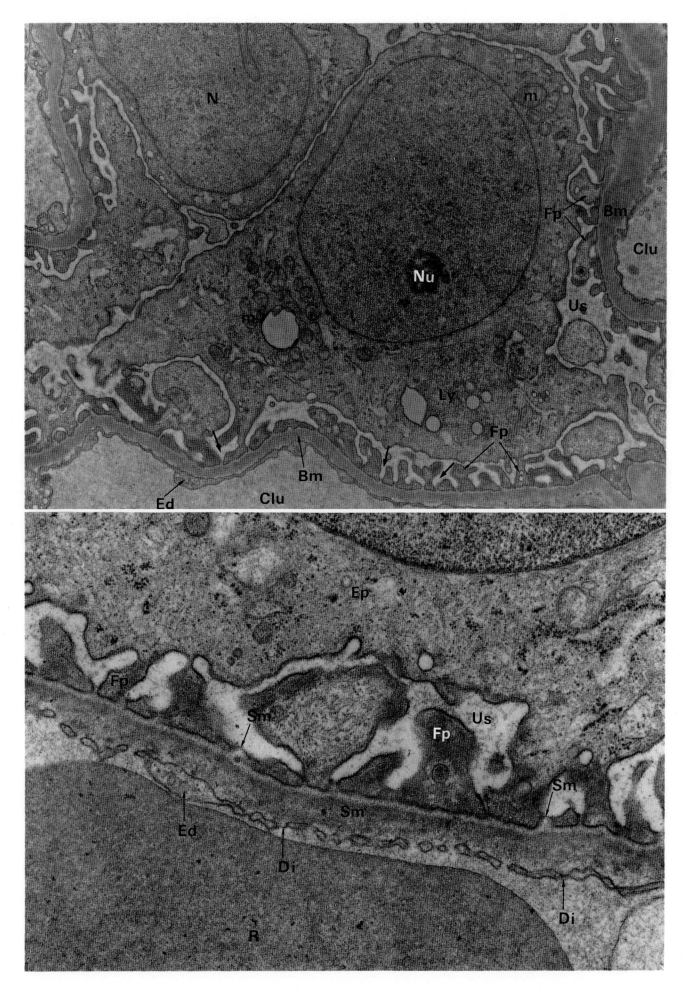

Macula densa and polkissen of the juxtaglomerular apparatus

The macula densa (Md) is a specialized part of the distal tubule located at the vascular pole of the glomerulus. The epithelial cells of this part are taller in height than those of other portions of the distal tubule. The cells have an ovoid nucleus located in their center. Their irregular free surface has a few small microvilli and single cilium (Cil). The space between the adjacent cells is dilated near the cell base and forms an extracellular compartment (Ec) which is filled with dense material. The basal cell membrane exhibits complex interdigitations. Numerous mitochondria (m) and a few strands of granular endoplasmic reticulum (Er) are contained in the supra- and infranuclear cytoplasm. Golgi complexes (Go) occur lateral to the nucleus. Some dense bodies (Db) are scattered throughout the cytoplasm.

Cells of the polkissen (Lc) are irregular in shape and have peripheral cytoplasmic processes. Their cytoplasm contains an inconspicuous endoplasmic reticulum, a few mitochondria and one or two small cytoplasmic granules (Gr) similar to those seen in the epitheloid cells in the wall of the afferent arteriole.

BBm: Basement membrane of Bowman's capsule.
Bl: Basal lamina beneath the macula densa.
Ep: Epithelial cell of glomerulus.
Lp: Lipofuscin pigment.
Tlu: Tubular lumen.

Material and method are the same as those of the picture on page 179.   ×5,000.

REFERENCE:

Biava, C. G. and M. West: Fine structure of normal human juxtaglomerular cells. I. General structure and intercellular relationships. Amer. J. Pathol., *49*: 679-721, 1966.

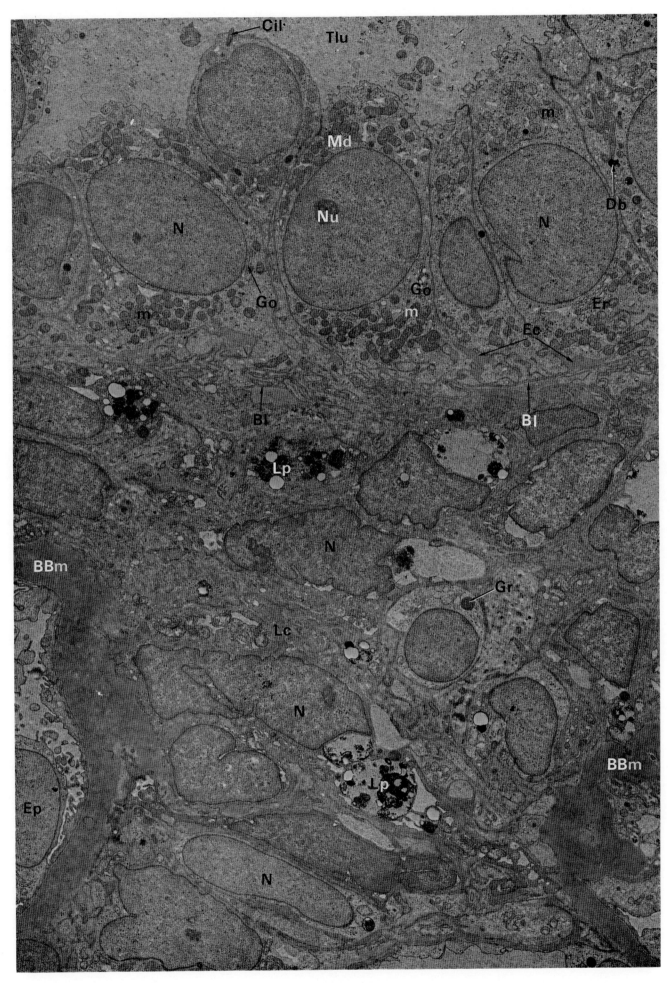

187

Epithelial cell of the proximal convoluted tubule

The proximal convolution is the part of the renal tubule where the reabsorption of water, glucose, sodium chloride and other substances takes place vigorously. The apical surface of the epithelial cell is provided with numerous microvilli (Mv). In the cytoplasm beneath the microvilli, a number of pinocytotic invaginations (Iv) and vesicles (v) are seen. Absorption droplets (Ad), limited by a membrane sac, occur in the supranuclear area. Mitochondria (m) of large size are scattered throughout the cytoplasm. The basal cytoplasm is apparently divided into small compartments (Sc) limited by a double membrane. This structure is thought to be formed as the result of complex lateral interdigitations between adjacent cells.

Bl : Basal lamina.
Go : Golgi complex.
Jc : Junctional complex.
N : Nucleus.
Nu : Nucleolus.
Tlu : Tubular lumen.

Material and method are the same as those of the picture on page 179. ×11,500.

REFERENCES :

ERICSSON, J. L. E., A. BERGSTRAND, G. ANDRES, H. BUCHT and G. CINOTTI: Morphology of the renal tubular epithelium in young, healthy humans. Acta path. microbiol. scand., *63*: 361–384, 1965.

TISCHER, C. C., R. E. BULGER, and B. F. TRUMP: Human renal ultrastructure. I. Proximal tubule of healthy individuals. Lab. Invest., *15*: 1357–1394, 1966.

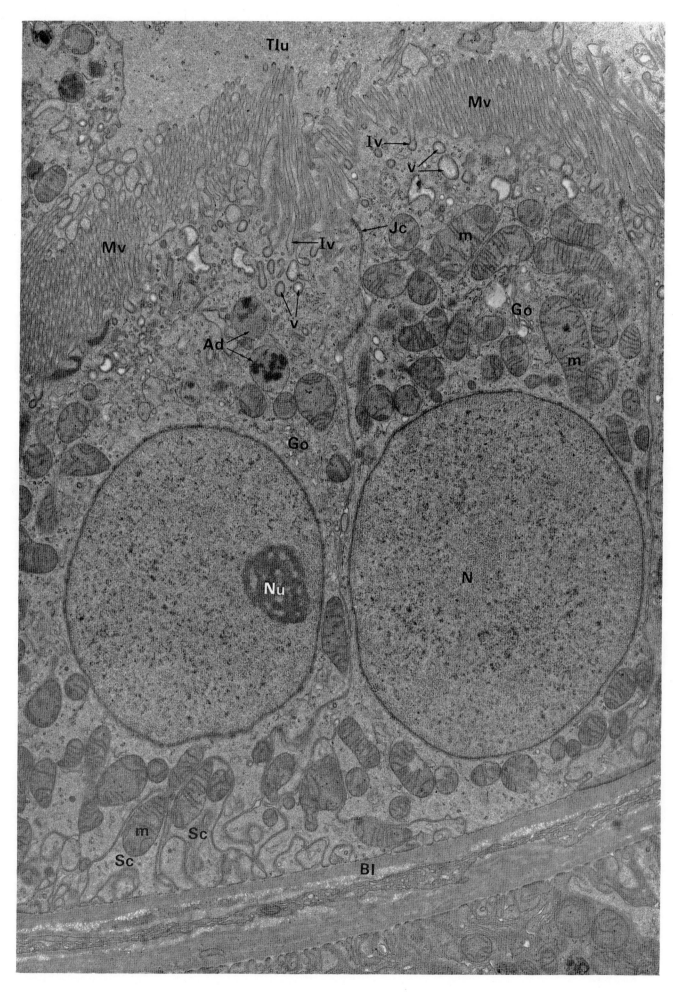

189

Epithelial cell of the distal convoluted tubule

The distal convolution is the part of the renal tubule where water is reabsorbed under the influence of an antidiuretic hormone (ADH). Replaced by potassium, hydrogen and ammonia, sodium is also removed from the urine in this portion of the tubule, resulting in acidification of the urine.

The epithelial cells of the distal convolution are a truncated pyramid in shape, demonstrating a convex luminal surface. A large ovoid nuclus (N) locates relatively high in the cell. The cell surface shows a few short, blunt microvilli (Mv). Lateral cell membranes are interdigitated near the cell base. Golgi complexes (Go) usually occur around the nucleus. Mitochondria (m) of highly variable profiles are numerously scattered all over the cytoplasm. Smooth- and rough-surfaced endoplasmic reticulum, in the form of vesicles, and free ribosomes are seen throughout the cytoplasm. The cell further contains numerous dense bodies (Db), some of which have internal fine granules, and some lipofuscin pigments (Lp). The capillary endothelium (Ed) is fenestrated.

Bl : Basal lamina.
Clu : Capillary lumen.
Id : Interdigitation of lateral cell membranes.
Jc : Junctional complex.
Tlu : Tubular lumen.

Material and method are the same as those of the picture on page 179.　×11,500.

REFERENCE:

Tisher, C. C., R. E. Bulger and B. F. Trump: Human renal ultrastructure. III. The distal tubule in healthy individuals. Lab. Invest., *18*: 655–668, 1968.

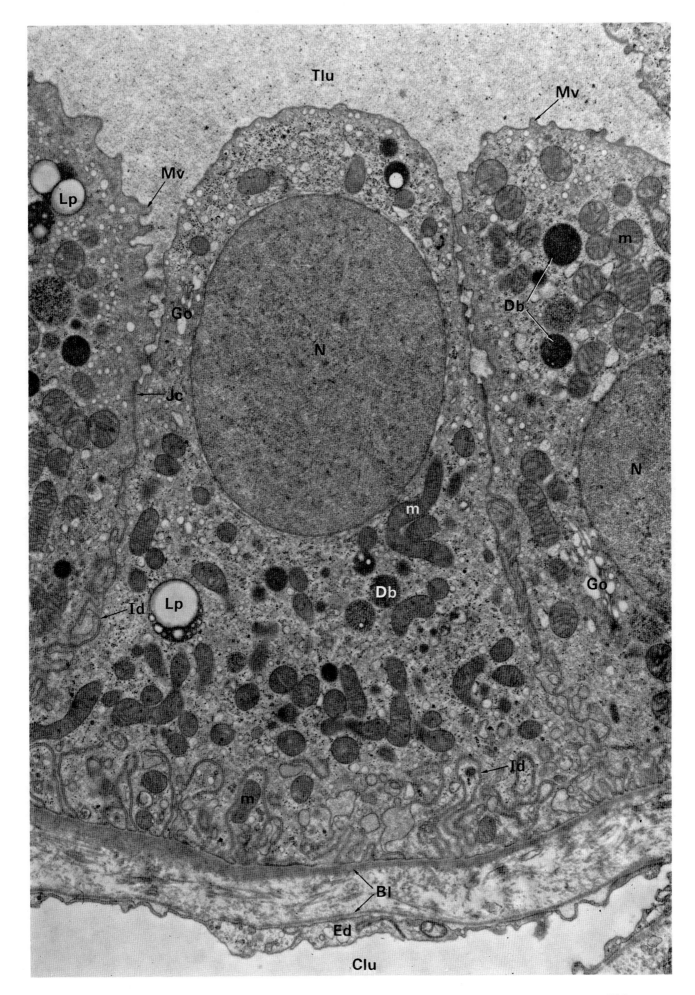

191

Apical surface of the proximal tubule epithelium (Top)

The luminal surface of the epithelial cells of the proximal convolution is covered by closely-arranged slender microvilli (Mv). Invaginations (Iv) of the surface cell membrane between the bases of the microvilli and the consequent vesicles (v) are considered to be a morphological equivalence of the tubular reabsorption by micropinocytosis. Vacuoles (Va) containing a few vesicles also occur in the apical cytoplasm.

Ad: Absorption droplet.
Jc: Junctional complex.

Basal portion of the distal tubule epithelium (Bottom)

The lateral surface membranes of the adjacent cells show such an elaborate interdigitation near the cell base that the basal cytoplasm appears divided into small compartments (Sc) limited by cell membranes in which large elongate mitochondria (m) are packed. Mitochondria are also numerous in the infranuclear cytoplasm.

Bl: Basal lamina.
Go: Golgi complex.
N: Nucleus.

Top and Bottom: Material and method are the same as those of the picture on page 179. Top: ×27,000. Bottom: ×20,000.

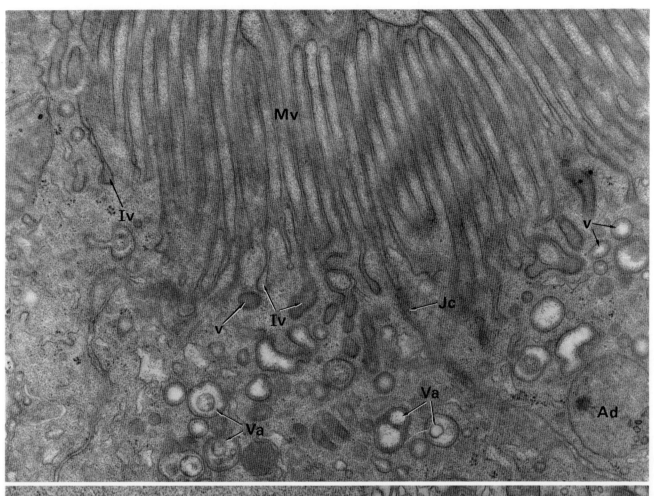

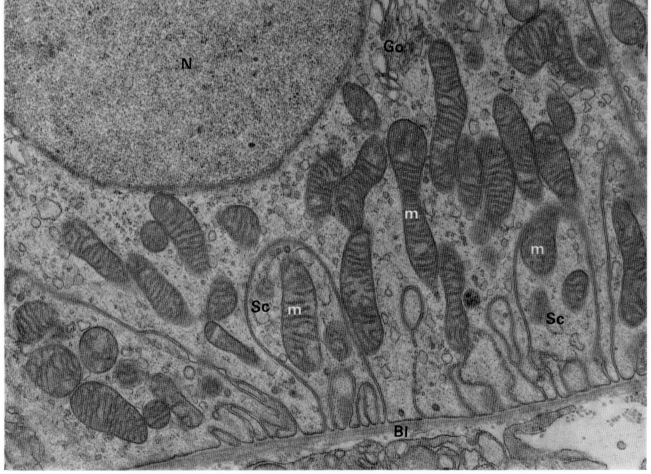

Epithelial cell of the collecting tubule

The collecting tubule is lined by a cuboidal epithelium. In this micrograph two types of epithelial cells, light and dark, are distinguishable. The outline of both types of cells is similar. The apical surface membrane is irregular, and a few small, blunt microvilli (Mv) are present at its margin. Lateral cell membranes show prominent interdigitations (Id) between adjacent cells. The light cell (Lc) has a central round nucleus with a prominent nucleolus (Nu). Small and spherical mitochondria (m) are scattered throughout the cytoplasm. Dense bodies (Db) are present in the apical cytoplasm. The infoldings of the basal cell membrane are slightly developed. The dark cell (Dc), also called intercalated cell, is similar to the epithelial cell of the distal convolution. The cell appears dark due to a large number of free ribosomes filling the cytoplasm. Numerous vesicles are also contained within the whole cytoplasm. The capillary seen in the interstitium is lined by fenestrated endothelial cells (Ed). The highly concentrated urine is made while passing through the collecting tubule, the wall of which becomes permeable to water in the presence of ADH.

Bl: Basal lamina.
c: Centriole.
Clu: Capillary lumen.
Jc: Junctional complex.
N: Nucleus.
PT: Epithelium of the proximal tubule.
Tlu: Tubular lumen.

Material and method are the same as those of the picture on page 179.　×10,000.

REFERENCE:

Myers, C. H., R. E. Bulger, C. C. Tisher and B. F. Trump: Human renal ultrastructure. IV. Collecting duct of healthy individuals. Lab. Invest., *15*: 1921–1950, 1966.

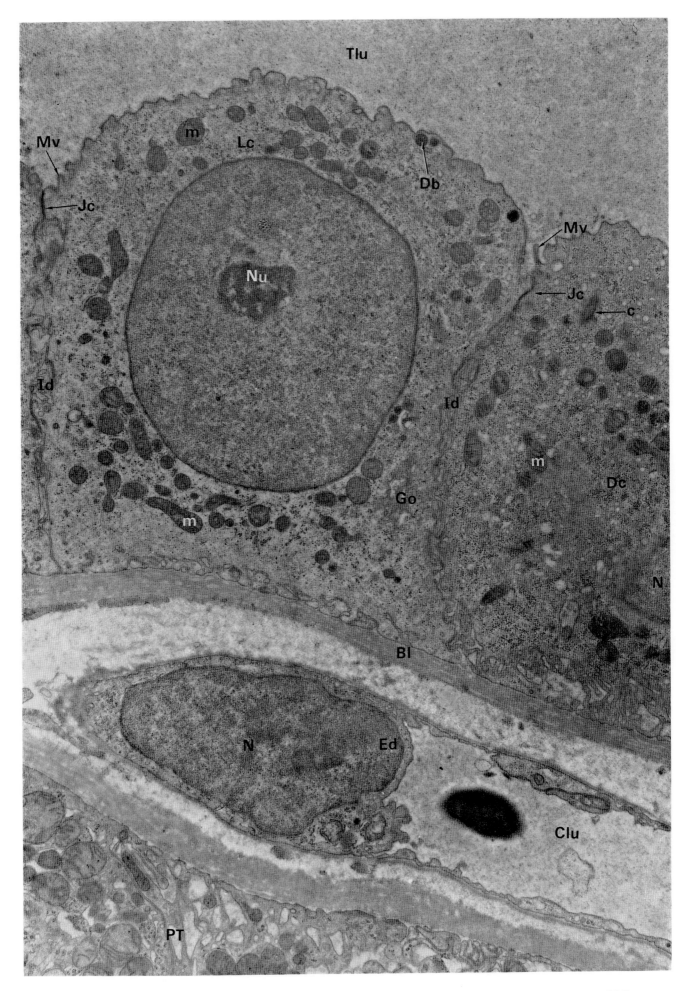

Transitional epithelium of the urinary bladder

The transitional epithelium lines the excretory passage of the urinary system from the renal calyces to the urethra which undergoes great changes in surface area as a result of contraction and dilation of the wall. This type of epithelium was previously believed to be a transitional form between the stratified squamous and stratified columnar epithelia. On the basis of his observation using polarization microscopy, Tanaka (1962) revealed that all cells of the transitional epithelium are in contact with the basal lamina; thus, the transitional epithelium is a kind of pseudostratified epithelium. His assumption was supported by an electron microscopic study by Petry and Amon (1966).

With the exception of the surface by which they attach themselves to the basal lamina (Bl), all transitional epithelial cells are entirely covered by numerous microvilli. The cytoplasm contains numerous mitochondria (m), small Golgi complexes, lysosomes (Ly), numerous free ribosomes and abundant tonofilaments. The intercellular space (Is) is wide and seems to form a three-dimensional network of canalicules which apparently extend from the basal lamina to the luminal surface where the space is sealed by a junctional complex. The lateral surfaces of adjacent cells are frequently attached by desmosomes.

Characteristic thick-walled vesicles are reported in the transitional epithelial cells of rodents such as the rat and the mouse. It is said that they may be structures for storage of the cell membrane of the transitional epithelial cells. However, there seems to be a great species variation in these vesicles. In the human transitional epithelial cell they are, if present, not so prominent as in the rodent transitional epithelium.

        Ed :   Capillary endothelium.
        Lu :   Lumen.
        N :   Nucleus.
        Nu :   Nucleolus.
        R :   Erythrocyte.

This material was obtained from the uninvolved area around the bladder tumor of a 63-year-old male. Cacodylate-buffered 2.5% glutaraldehyde fixation followed by post-fixation with 2.0% osmium tetroxide solution. Stained with lead tartarate. ×3,300.

REFERENCES :

TANAKA, K.: Polarisationsoptische Analyse der Übergangsepithelien des Menschen. Arch. histol. jap., *22*: 229-236, 1962.

PETRY, G. und H. AMON: Licht- und electronenmikroskopische Studien über Struktur und Dynamik des Übergangsepithels. Z. Zellforsch., *69*: 587-612, 1966.

MONIS, B. and D. ZAMBRANO: Ultrastructure of transitional epithelium of man. Z. Zellforsch., *87*: 101-117, 1968.

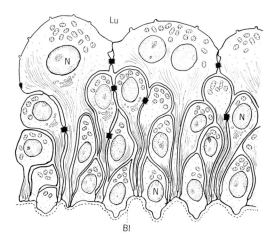

A diagram showing the fine structure of the transitional epithelium.

        Bl :   Basal lamina.
        Lu :   Lumen.
        N :   Nucleus.

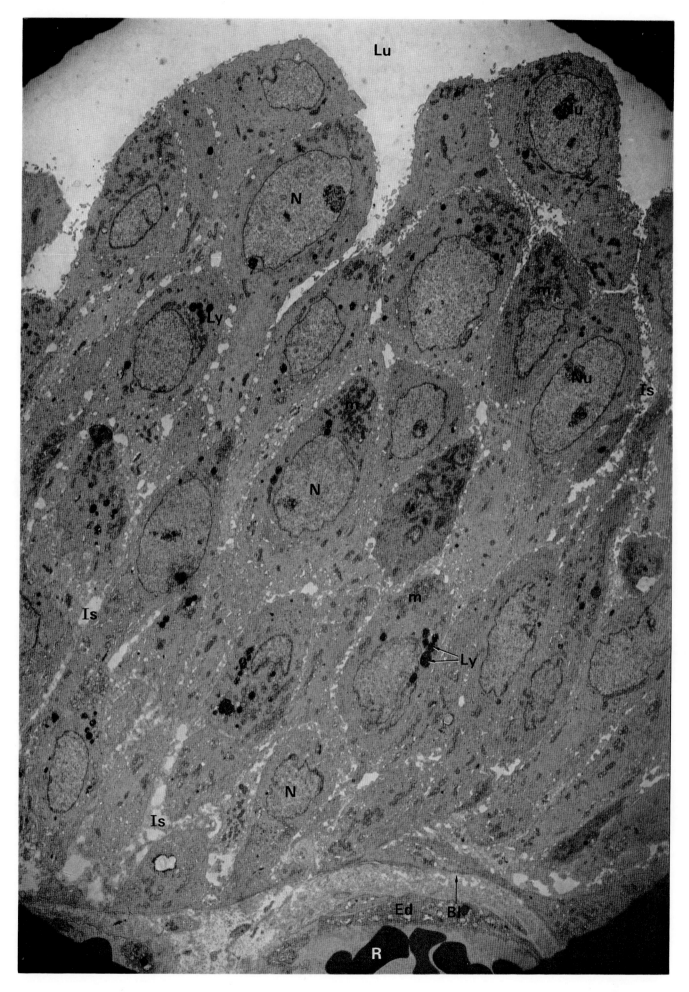

The parenchyme of the human testis consists of seminiferous tubules and interstitial cells filling the spaces between the tubules. The seminiferous tubules are, for the most part, conspicuously convoluted and measure up to 200 m in their total length. In the basal part of the convoluted tubules we can see the youngest representatives of the spermatogenetic cells supported by the cytoplasm of Sertoli cells.

Seminiferous tubule (Top)

Two spermatogonia (Sg), a primary spermatocyte (Psc) and two Sertoli cells (Sc) are seen. The cytoplasm of the primary spermatocyte is richer and less dense than that of the spermatogonium. Sertoli cells have ample cytoplasm containing lipofuscin granules (Lp) and large lipid droplets (Ld). The peritubular connective tissue (Pct) consists of several layers of slender cytoplasmic processes of fibrocytes.

N: Nucleus.
Nu: Nucleolus.

Spermatogonium (Bottom)

The spermatogonium is the most primitive spermatogenic cell. It increases in number by normal mitotic division and gives rise to the primary spermatocyte. In this electron micrograph, two spermatogonia, probably A type (Sg), resting upon the basal lamina (Bl), are shown. The cells of this type are already combined with each other by an intercellular bridge (arrow). Note the local thickening of the plasma membrane covering the bridge and the microtubules passing through the latter.

Cf: Collagenous fiber.
Go: Golgi complex.
Lc: Lubarsch's crystalloid.
m: Mitochondrion.
Sc: Sertoli cell.
Va: Vacuoles of unknown nature.
*: Infolding of the basement membrane.

Top and Bottom: Biopsy material obtained for diagnostic purpose from a 27-year-old sterile male. Phosphate-buffered glutaraldehyde fixation followed by post-fixation with 1.3% osmium tetroxide solution. Doubly stained with uranyl acetate and lead tartarate. Top: ×4,000. Bottom: ×6,300. (Photographs courtesy of Dr. Y. Togawa)

REFERENCES:

Clermont, Y.: Cycle of the seminiferous epithelium in man. Amer. J. Anat., *112*: 35–51, 1963.

Togawa, Y.: Occurrence and structure of intercellular bridges between the human spermatogonia. Arch. histol. jap., *33*: 301–317, 1971.

Tres, L. L. and A. J. Solari: The ultrastructure of the nuclei and the behaviour of the sex chromosomes of human spermatogonia. Z. Zellforsch., *91*: 75–89, 1968.

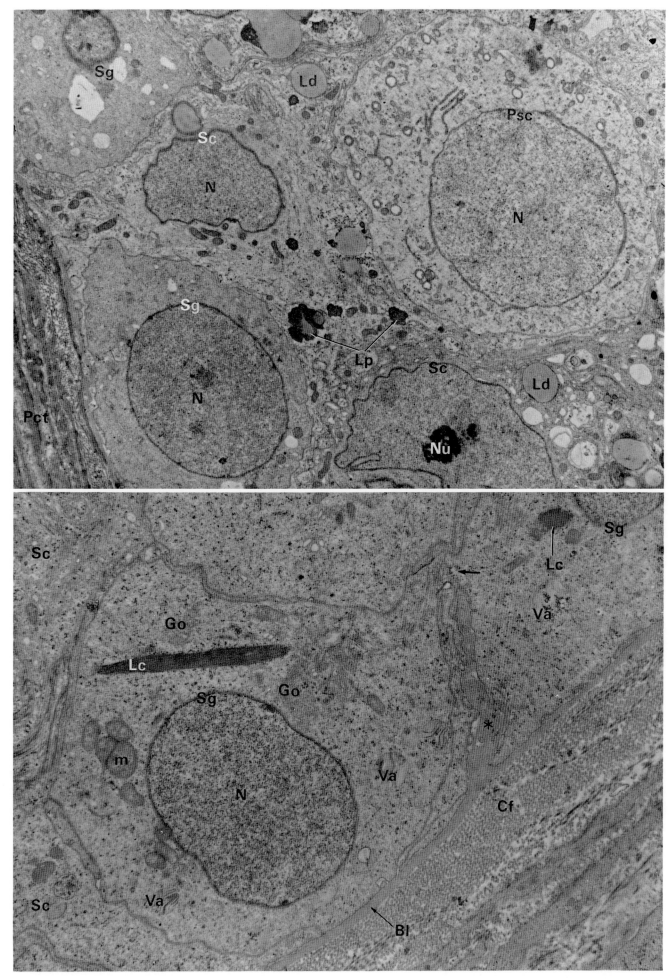

Sertoli cell (Top)

The Sertoli cell is the supporting and nutritive element of the seminiferous tubule to which the spermatid attaches during its transformation period. Human Sertoli cells are characterized by the occurrence of Charcot-Böttcher's crystalloid (C-Bc).

In this picture, basal portions of three Sertoli cells are seen. The nucleus has a deep indentation at the arrow and the karyoplasm is relatively homogeneous except for a large, prominent nucleolus (Nu). The cytoplasm contains granular endoplasmic reticulum, free ribosomes, cytoplasmic filaments, microtubules and a number of slender mitochondria (m).

Bl : Basal lamina.
Go : Golgi complex.
Ld : Lipid droplet.

Testis of a 26-year-old sterile male. Method is the same as the pictures on page 199. ×5,400.

Primary spermatocyte (Bottom)

The primary spermatocyte is the largest cell among spermatogenic cells. Like usual somatic cells, it has 46 chromosomes. However, the division which occurs in the primary spermatocyte is a reduction division, or meiosis, resulting in the formation of secondary spermatocytes having half of the chromosomes. The secondary spermatocyte is short-lived and soon divides mitotically to produce spermatids.

In the nucleus of the primary spermatocyte shown in this electron micrograph at least four synaptonemal complexes (arrows) are seen, each of which consists of two lateral elements and a central element. The nucleolus (Nu) is large and prominent. In the lower left corner two mature spermatids are seen attaching themselves to the cytoplasm of the Sertoli cell.

Go : Golgi complex.
m : Mitochondrion.
Sc : Sertoli cell.
Spz : Mature spermatid.

Operatively obtained testis of a 17-year-old male with hydrocele testis. Method is the same as that of the pictures on page 199. ×8,600. (Photographs courtesy of Dr. Y. TOGAWA)

REFERENCES :

BAWA, S. R. : Fine structure of the Sertoli cell of the human testis. J. Ultrastr. Res., *9*: 459-474, 1963.

NAGANO, T. : Some observations on the fine structure of the Sertoli cell in the human testis. Z. Zellforsch., *73*: 89-106, 1966.

TRES, L. L. and A. J. SOLARI : The ultrastructure of the human sex vesicle. Chromosoma, *22*: 16-31, 1967.

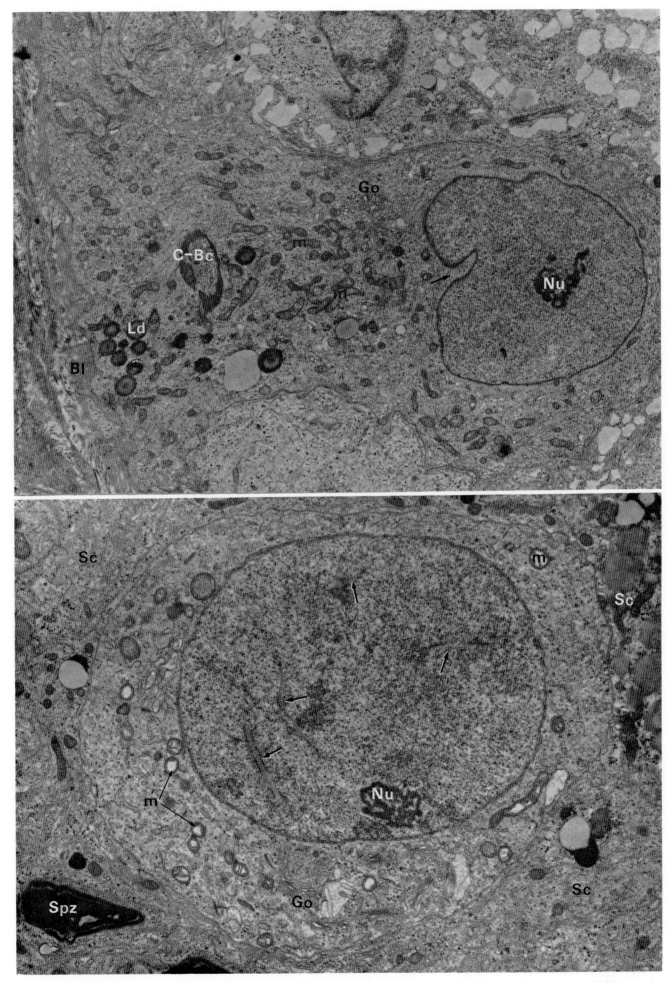

Spermatid

The daughter cells of the secondary spermatocytes are the spermatids in which cell division no longer occurs. They transform into mature spermatozoa by a complicated cytological process called spermiogenesis, which has many points still to be elucidated.

Top: The spermatid shown in this figure has a large oval nucleus (N) which is located in the center of the cell and contains moderately electron opaque karyoplasm. In the cytoplasm there are several mitochondria (m) and scattered profiles of agranular endoplasmic reticulum. Approximately one-third of the nuclear surface is covered by an acrosomal vesicle (arrows), in which a large acrosomal granule (Ag) is contained. Cisterns and vesicles of the Golgi complex (Go) are closely associated with the outer surface of the acrosomal vesicle.

Sc: Sertoli cell.

Bottom: Spermatids at an advanced stage of spermiogenesis. The nucleus (N) is somewhat polygonal in shape and contains granular karyoplasm of medium density. One pole of the nucleus is covered by an acrosomal cap (Ac) filled with dense material and is closely applied to the cell membrane. At the opposite pole of the nucleus there is a pair of centrioles. One of these is called the transverse centriole (Cet) and the other is the longitudinal centriole (Cel) which gives rise to the axial filament (Af). The latter is surrounded by a thin cytoplasmic sheath which is separated from the adjoining cytoplasm by a membrane cleft (arrows). From the posterior end of the acrosomal cap microtubules extend caudally to form the manchette (Ma). Several mitochondria (m) are seen, but they do not as yet aggregate around the axial filament to form the middle piece. A chromatoid body (Ch) occurs also in the cytoplasm. Note the intercellular bridge (*) connecting the two spermatids through which the spermatids develop synchronously. Around the spermatids are seen a primary spermatocyte (Ps), portions of Sertoli cells (Sc) and cross sections of the tail of mature spermatozoa (Ts).

Top and Bottom: Testis surgically obtained from a 17-year-old male with hydrocele testis. Method is the same as that of the pictures on page 199. Top and Bottom: ×11,000. (Photographs courtesy of Dr. Y. Togawa)

REFERENCES:

Horstmann, E.: Elektronenmikroskopische Untersuchungen zur Spermiohistogenese beim Menschen, Z. Zellforsch., *54*: 68–89, 1961.
Clermont, Y.: The cycle of the seminiferous epithelium in man. Amer. J. Anat., *112*: 35–51, 1963.
De Kretser, D. M.: Ultrastructural features of human spermiogenesis. Z. Zellforsch., *98*: 477–505, 1969.

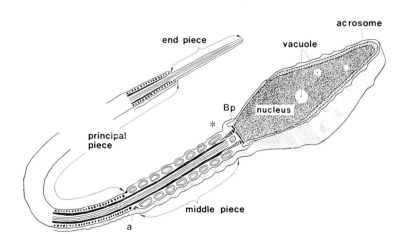

A schematic drawing of a mature spermatozoon.
a: Annulus.
Bp: Basal plate.
*: Centriole.
(Courtesy of Dr. T. Fujita)

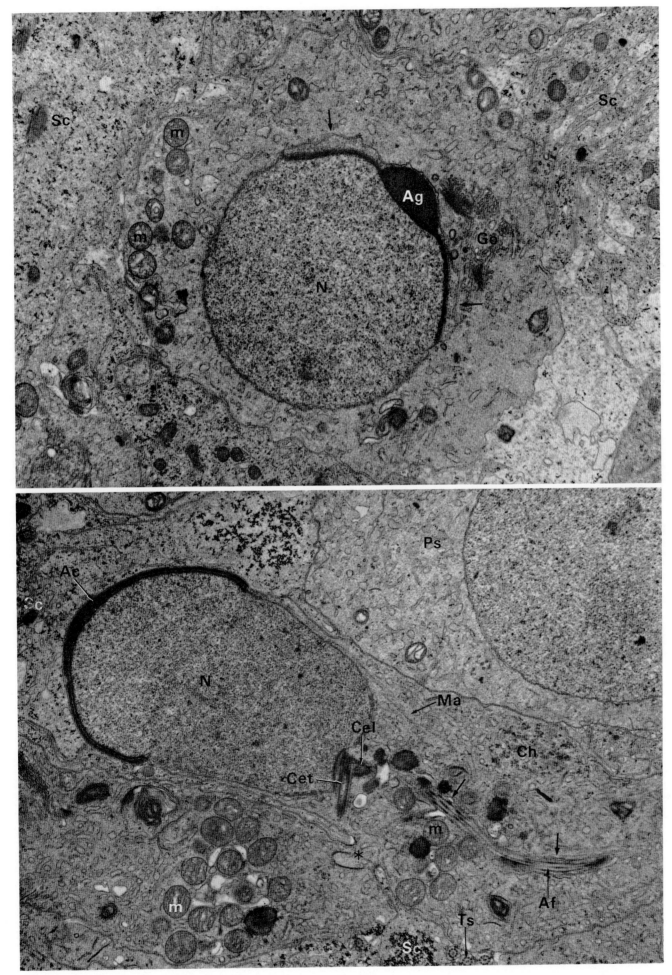

203

Spermatozoon

The human spermatozoon is characterized by an oval and flattened shape of the head. The tail contains the axial core consisting of microtubules which show a characteristic 9-plus-2 pattern essentially identical to that in the cilium. It is, as in other mammalian species, usually divided into three portions: middle piece, principal piece and end piece. The axial core and associated row of coarse, dense fibers (Df) are surrounded in the middle piece by a characteristic mitochondrial sheath (m) and in the principal piece by a dense, concentrically oriented fibrous sheath. No specialized sheath is seen in the end piece.

1. A survey picture of an ejaculated spermatozoon. This spermatozoon is immature as it still has a cytoplasmic droplet (Cd). This is a remnant of the cytoplasm in the spermatid. Although normal human ejaculate contains a certain number of immature spermatozoa, there are sterilities due to an abundance of them. Note that the coarse, dense fibers do not continue directly to the segmented column, but attach from inside to the latter (arrow).

> Ac: Acrosomal cap.
> N: Nucleus.
> Nm: Nuclear envelope.

2. Longitudinal section through the neck portion.

> Bp: Basal plate.
> *: Proximal centriole.

3. Longitudinal section through the caudal end of the middle piece and beginning of the principal piece.

> a: Annulus.

4. Cross section through the head cap.

> Ac: Acrosomal cap.
> Cm: Cell membrane.
> N: Nucleus.
> Sas: Subacrosomal space.

5. Cross section of the middle piece.
6, 7. Cross section of the principal piece at two different levels.
8. Cross section through the end piece.

All photographs shown in this plate were obtained from the ejaculate of a 36-year-old male of proved normal fertility. Phosphate-buffered 1.0% glutaraldehyde fixation followed by post-fixation with 1.0% osmium tetroxide solution. Uranyl acetate and lead tartarate staining. 1. ×16,000. 2. ×80,000. 3. ×60,000. 4–8. ×40,000. (Photographs courtesy of Dr. M. MIYOSHI)

REFERENCES:

PEDERSEN, H.: Ultrastructure of the ejaculated human sperm. Z. Zellforsch., *94*: 542–554, 1969.

FUJITA, T., M. MIYOSHI and J. TOKUNAGA: Scanning and transmission electron microscopy of human ejaculate spermatozoa with special reference to their abnormal forms. Z. Zellforsch., *105*: 483–497, 1970.

ZAMBONI, L., R. ZEMJANIS and M. STEFANINI: The fine structure of monkey and human spermatozoa. Anat. Rec., *169*: 129–154, 1971.

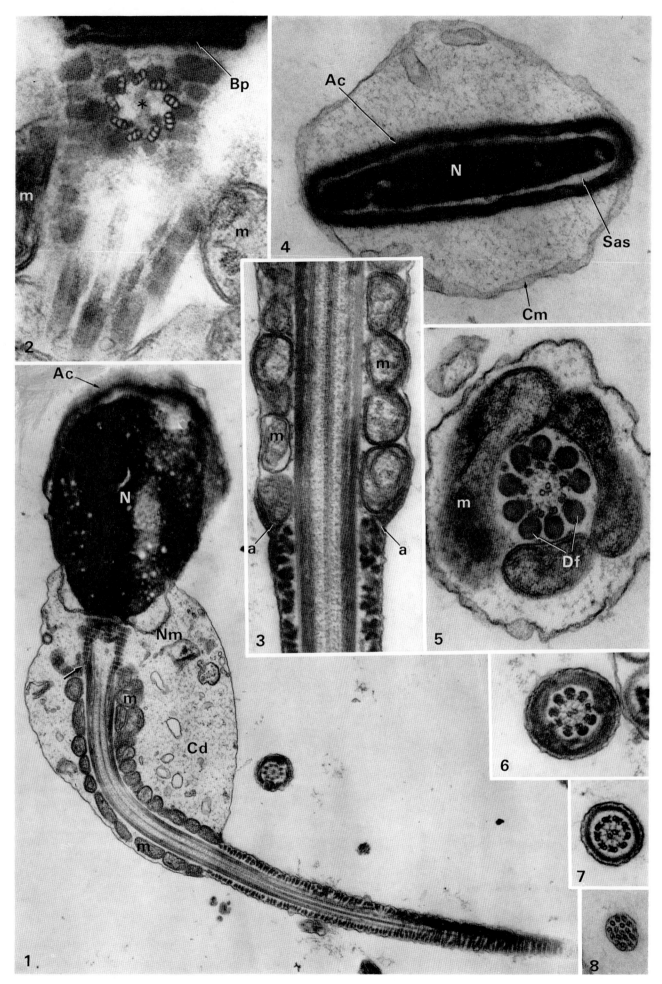

205

Interstitial cell

Top :   The interstitial cell of the testis, unlike most endocrine cells of epithelial origin, develops from a mesenchymal stroma and is located among the connective tissue elements between seminiferous tubules.   It furnishes the male sex hormone, testosterone.

The nucleus is round and large and contains a prominent nucleolus (Nu).   In this electron micrograph, an unique inclusion body (Inc) is seen in the karyoplasm, though it is not a constant structure.   The rich cytoplasm contains Golgi complexes (Go), mitochondria (m) and markedly-developed agranular endoplasmic reticulum.   The extensive occurrence of agranular endoplasmic reticulum generally characterizes the steroid-secreting cells and it is considered the site of steroid hormone production.   The vesicular appearance of agranular endoplasmic reticulum in this and the bottom pictures may be due to unfavorable fixation of the material: in ideally fixed material the agranular endoplasmic reticulum appears like a three-dimensional lattice-work of fine tubules as shown in the adrenal cortex.   The cytoplasm also contains lipid droplets (Ld) and numerous lysosomes (Ly).

Biopsy material obtained for diagnostic purpose from a 31-year-old sterile male. Phosphate-buffered 2.5% glutaraldehyde fixation followed by post-fixation with 1.3% osmium tetroxide solution.   Uranyl acetate and lead tartarate staining.   ×4,700.

Bottom :   Electron micrograph showing a part of an interstitial cell containing a peripheral portion of a nucleus (N), profiles of agranular endoplasmic reticulum, as well as crystalloid of Reinke in which a fine and regular structure is apparent.   The latter is characteristic of human interstitial cells, but its function remains obscure at present.   Fine filamentous material (arrows) seen between the vesicular agranular endoplasmic reticulum is believed to be a precursor of the crystalloid of Reinke.

        m :   Mitochondrion.
        Rc :   Reinke's crystalloid.
        ∗ :   Nuclear pore.

From the testis of a 53-year-old male with prostatic cancer.   Obtained by operation.   The method for specimen preparation is the same as that of the top picture.   ×44,000.   (Photograph courtesy of Dr. Y. Togawa)

REFERENCES :

Fawcett, D. W. and M. H. Burgos : Studies on the fine structure of the mammalian testis. II. The human interstitial tissue. Amer. J. Anat., *107* : 245–269, 1960.

Yamada, E. : Some observations on the fine structure of the interstitial cell in the human testis as revealed by electron microscopy. Gumma Symposia on Endocrinol., *2* : 1–17, 1965.

De Kretser, D. M. : The fine structure of the testicular interstitial cells in man of normal androgenic status. Z. Zellforsch., *80* : 594–609, 1967.

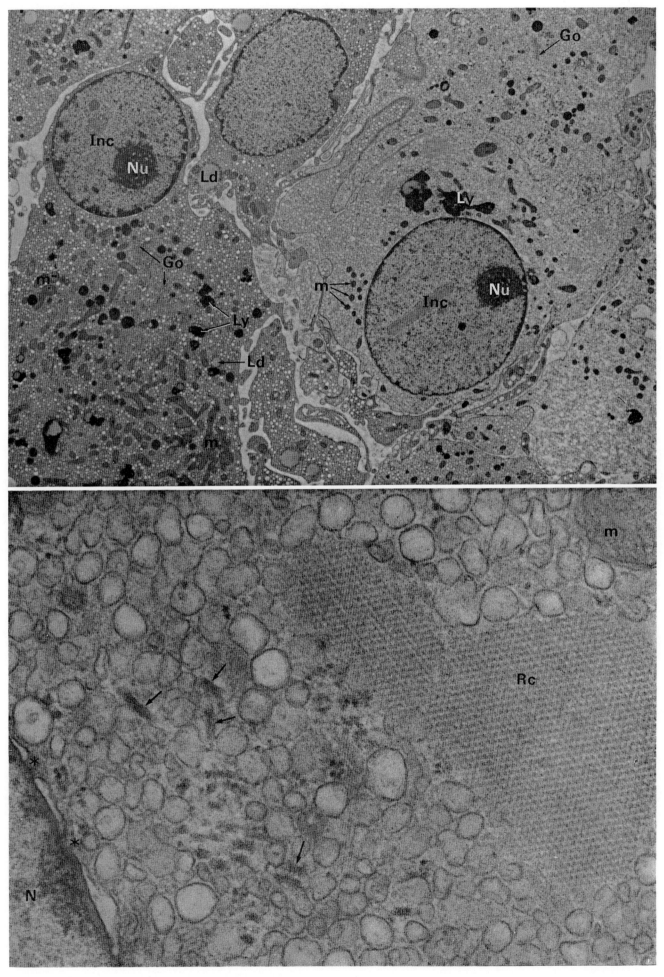

Glandular epithelium of the prostate

The prostate gland produces a major part of the seminal plasma. The glandular secretory epithelium of the prostate is normally simple columnar, but varies in height. Though microvilli (Mv) are usually provided on the free surface, they differ markedly in number from cell to cell. The lateral cell borders exhibit extensive pleated foldings (Id) which are elaborately interdigitated near the cell base with adjacent cells. The nucleus (N), with a prominent nucleolus (Nu), is located basally. In the supranuclear cytoplasm are seen numerous secretory vacuoles (Va) containing dense granular materials. These vacuoles finally accumulate toward the cell apex, so that the free surface of the cell becomes domed with few microvilli (arrow). It is suggested that the apical cytoplasm may be detached as secretory materials in the form of apocrine secretion. Large Golgi complexes (Go) occur in the supranuclear cytoplasm. Dense bodies (Db) and lipofuscin pigments are contained in small number. The basal cells (Bc) are located between the secretory cells and the basal lamina (Bl). They are one of the epithelial components constituting the prostate epithelia. A capillary (Cap) runs beneath the epithelium and some connective tissue elements intervene in between. The endothelial cell (Ed) lining the capillary is occasionally fenestrated.

d : Desmosome.
Fc : Fibrocyte.
Jc : Junctional complex.
Lu : Lumen.
Nl : Neutrophil leukocyte.
R : Erythrocyte.

Prostate of a 27-year-old male with bladder tumor. Obtained by surgical operation. Fixation with 2.0% osmium tetroxide in s-collidine buffer. Lead tartarate staining. ×8,700. (Photograph courtesy of Dr. K. Kano)

REFERENCE:

Brandes, D., D. Kirchheim and W. W. Scott: Ultrastructure of the human prostate. Normal and neoplastic. Lab. Invest., *13*: 1541–1560, 1964.

Fisher, E. R. and W. Jeffrey: Ultrastructure of human normal and neoplasmic prostate with comments relative to prostatic effects of hormonal stimulation in the rabbit. Amer. J. clin. Pathol., *44*: 119–134, 1965.

Mao, P. and A. Angrist: The fine structure of the basal cell of human prostate. Lab. Invest., *15*: 1768–1782, 1966.

Kirchheim, D. und R. L. Bacon : Elektronenmikroskopische Untersuchungen der normalen Prostata, der Prostata Hypertrophie und des Prostata-carcinoms. Urologe, *5*: 292–305, 1968.

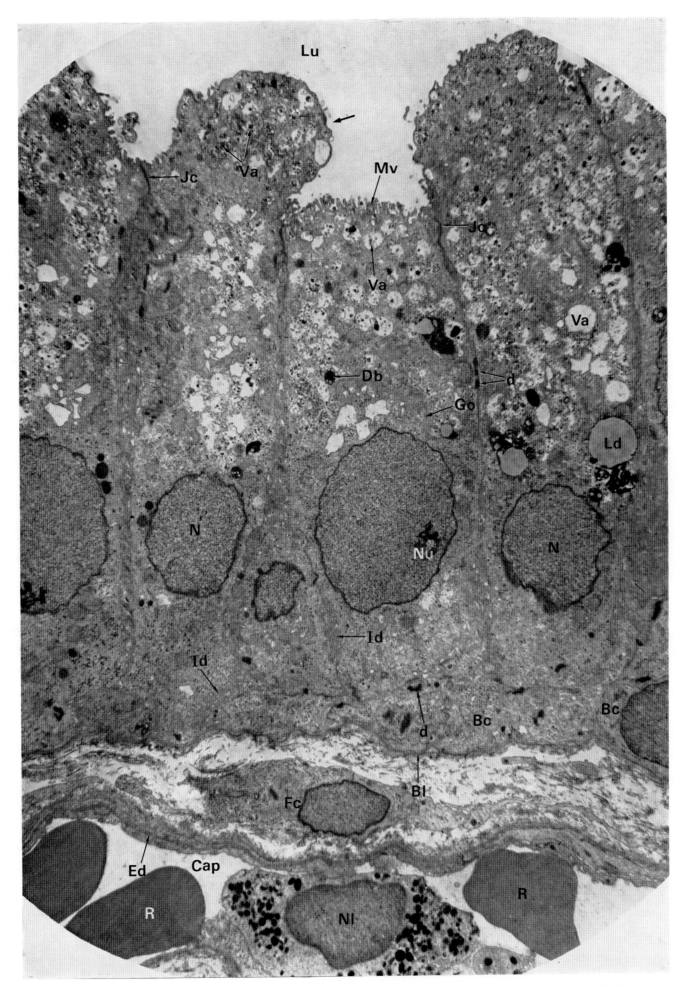

Germinal epithelium and tunica albuginea

The free surface of the ovary is covered by a specialized portion of the peritoneal epithelium which is called germinal epithelium because it was once believed to be the site of the origin of oogonia. However, it is now accepted that the primitive germ cells derived from the endoderm of the primitive yolk sac migrate into the ovary to become oogonia. Thus, the name germinal epithelium is only historical.

The cells composing this epithelium are cuboidal in shape and contain a small nucleus (N) of highly irregular contour with small nucleoli (Nu). A small number of long microvilli project from the luminal surface into the peritoneal cavity (Lu). The lateral surface of the epithelial cells is irregular and desmosomes occasionally occur here. The basal surface rests on the basal lamina (Bl) which separates the germinal epithelium from the connective tissue. The narrow cytoplasm of the epithelial cells contains small mitochondria (m), scarce endoplasmic reticulum and abundant cytoplasmic filaments and microtubules.

The connective tissue subjacent to the germinal epithelium consists, for the most part, of fibrocytes (Fc) and collagenous fibers (Cf), and is less vascularized and more compactly formed than the general stroma of the ovary. This layer is called tunica albuginea, because macroscopically it looks white.

Top: Survey picture of the germinal epithelium and the tunica albuginea (Ta). Collagenous fibrils in the tunica albuginea (Ta) are embedded in the dense matrix of the connective tissue so that they appear electron-lucent against a dark background.

Bottom: Detail of the cells of the germinal epithelium. The cytoplasm contains small mitochondria (m), lipid droplets (Ld), small Golgi complexes (Go) and a few elements of granular endoplasmic reticulum. The intercellular space is filled with dense amorphous material, the nature of which is not known.

Top and Bottom: From unaffected area around the surgically-removed ovarial cyst of a 31-year-old female. Phosphate-buffered 2.5% glutaraldehyde fixation followed by 1.0% osmium tetroxide post-fixation. Lead tartarate staining. Top: ×4,300. Bottom: ×15,500.

REFERENCE:

PAPADAKI, L. and J. O. W. BEILBY: The fine structure of the surface epithelium of the human ovary. J. Cell Sci., *8*: 445–465, 1971.

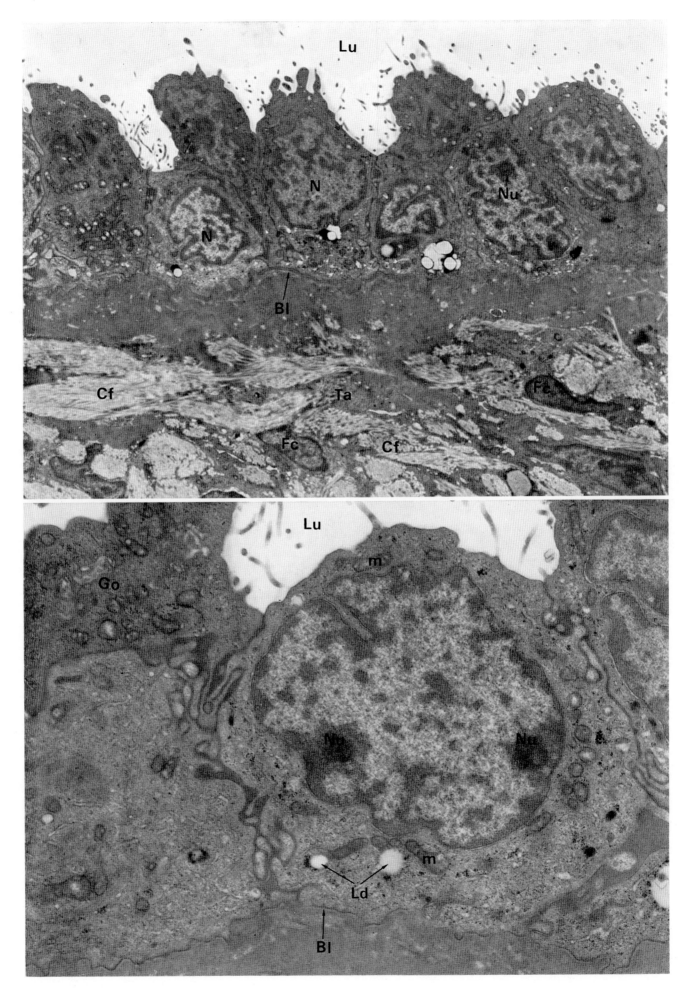

Primary oocyte

During fetal life, the oogonia increase in number by repeated cell divisions. Some of them become enlarged and are transformed into primary oocytes which are to undergo the first meiotic division.

Two electron micrographs of primary oocytes in the pachytene stage of prophase are shown here. The oocytes in this stage are characterized by nuclei containing so-called synaptonemal complexes. The synaptonemal complex consists of two lateral elements and a central one. This structure is said to represent two homologous chromosomes in close longitudinal union.

Top : Low-power electron micrograph showing primary oocytes in the pachytene stage surrounded by a layer of flattened follicle epithelial cells. The follicle epithelial cell (Foc) contains a dark, elongated nucleus. The nucleus of the oocyte is large, round and clear and limited by a nuclear envelope. A prominent nucleolus (Nu) is located in the periphery of the nucleus. The synaptonemal complexes are shown by arrows. The ample cytoplasm of the oocyte contains small, rounded mitochondria, profiles of Golgi complexes and a few strands of granular endoplasmic reticulum (Er). In the connective tissue space are seen a cross-sectioned blood capillary (Cap), profiles of fibroblasts (Fb) and bundles of collagenous fibrils.

Bottom : A portion of a primary oocyte in the pachytene stage. In the nucleus, a nucleolus (Nu) and profiles of synaptonemal complexes (arrows) are seen. The cytoplasm, separated from the nucleus by the nuclear envelope (Nm), contains rounded mitochondria (m) which have a few cristae. A Golgi complex (Go) and fine granular substances are also seen.

From the ovary of a 7-month fetus (♀, 800 g). Phosphate-buffered 2.5% glutaraldehyde fixation followed by 1.0% osmium tetroxide post-fixation. Lead tartarate staining. Top: ×3,000. Bottom: ×14,000.

REFERENCES:

BACA, M. and L. ZAMBONI: The fine structure of human follicular oocytes. J. Ultrastr. Res., *19*: 354–381, 1967.

BAKER, T. G. and L. L. FRANCHI: The fine structure of oogonia and oocytes in human ovaries. J. Cell Sci., *2*: 213–224, 1967.

GREEN, J. A. and M. MAQUEO: Ultrastructure of the human ovary. 1. The luteral cell during the menstrual cycle. Amer. J. Obstet. Gynecol., *92*: 946–957, 1965.

HERTIG, A. T. and E. C. ADAMS: Studies on the human oocytes and its follicle. 1. Ultrastructural and histochemical observations on the primordial follicle stage. J. Cell Biol., *34*: 647–675, 1967.

ZAMBONI, L., D. R. MISHELL, J. H. BELL and M. BACA: Fine structure of the human ovum in the pronuclear stage. J. Cell Biol., *30*: 579–600, 1966.

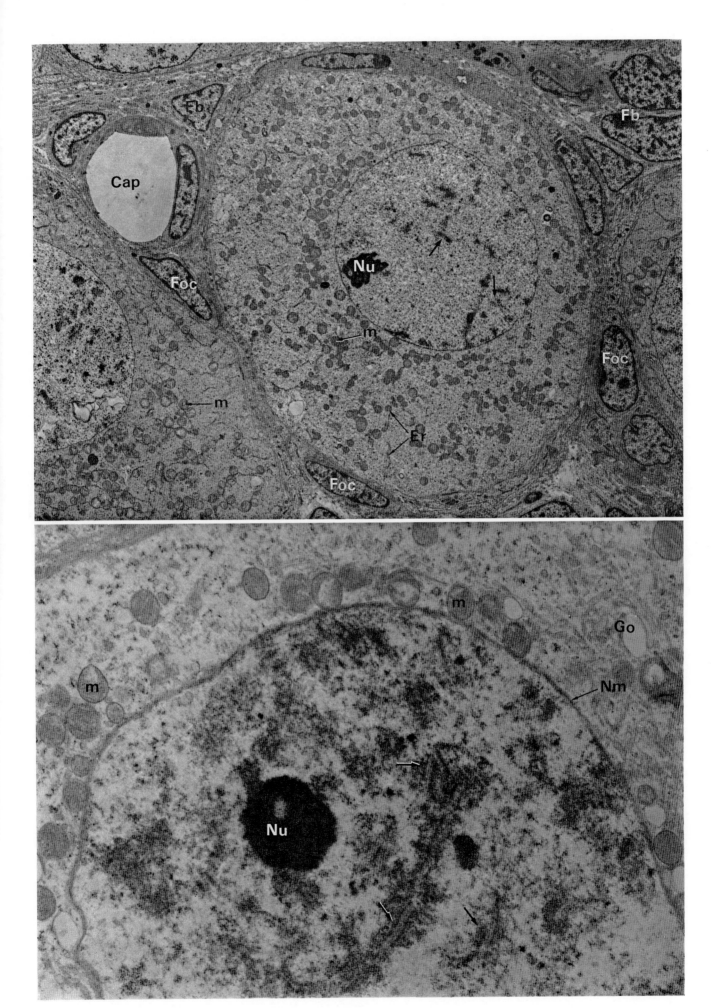

Primary follicle

The primary follicle is formed of a primary oocyte in the interphase surrounded by a single layer of follicle epithelial cells. In the first stage of development, the primary oocyte is relatively small and the follicle epithelial cells are flattened in shape. When the follicle begins to grow after puberty, the oocyte increases in size, the flattened follicular cells become cuboidal to low columnar and then, as a result of continued divisions, they become stratified.

Top : This micrograph shows a primary follicle in its early stages of growth. In the upper left corner is a portion of a nucleus (N) surrounded by a nuclear envelope (Nm). In the cytoplasm of the oocyte are seen abundant profiles of round mitochodria (m), large polymorphous lysosomes (Ly), a Golgi complex (Go), strands of endoplasmic reticulum (Er) and so forth. The follicular cells (Foc) surrounding the oocyte are cuboidal in shape and have roughly round nuclei. The basal surface of the follicular cells rests on a thick basement membrane (Bm). Spindle-shaped fibroblasts and bundles of collagenous fibrils are seen immediately surrounding the follicle.

Bottom : A closer view of the follicle epithelial cells and the basement membrane of the same follicle as that shown in the top picture. Most of the cell is occupied by a nucleus with deep indentations (In). The cytoplasm contains small mitochondria (m), a few strands of granular endoplasmic reticulum, filaments and free ribosomes. The basal and lateral cell surfaces are smooth. On the surface applying to that of the oocyte (Ov) there are a considerable number of microvillous projections (Mv). In the basement membrane (Bm), on which the follicular epithelial cells rest, are a number of parallel-arranged filaments which are considerably thinner than the collagenous fibrils (Cf) seen in the stroma.

> Ly: Lysosome.
> Nu: Nucleolus.

Top and Bottom : Surgically-obtained ovary of a 32-year-old female with carcinoma colli. Phosphate-buffered 2.5% glutaraldehyde fixation followed by 1.0% osmium tetroxide post-fixation. Uranyl acetate and lead tartarate staining. Top: ×3,800. Bottom: ×12,000.

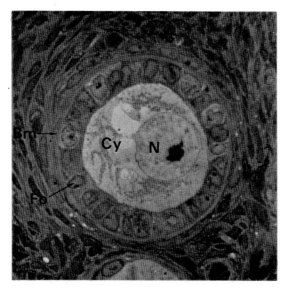

Photomicrograph of a primary follicle
Electron micrographs shown on page 215 were obtained from the same follicle. Stained with toluidine blue. ×700.

> N: Nucleus.
> Cy: Cytoplasm.
> Fo: Follicular cell layer.
> Bm: Basement membrane.

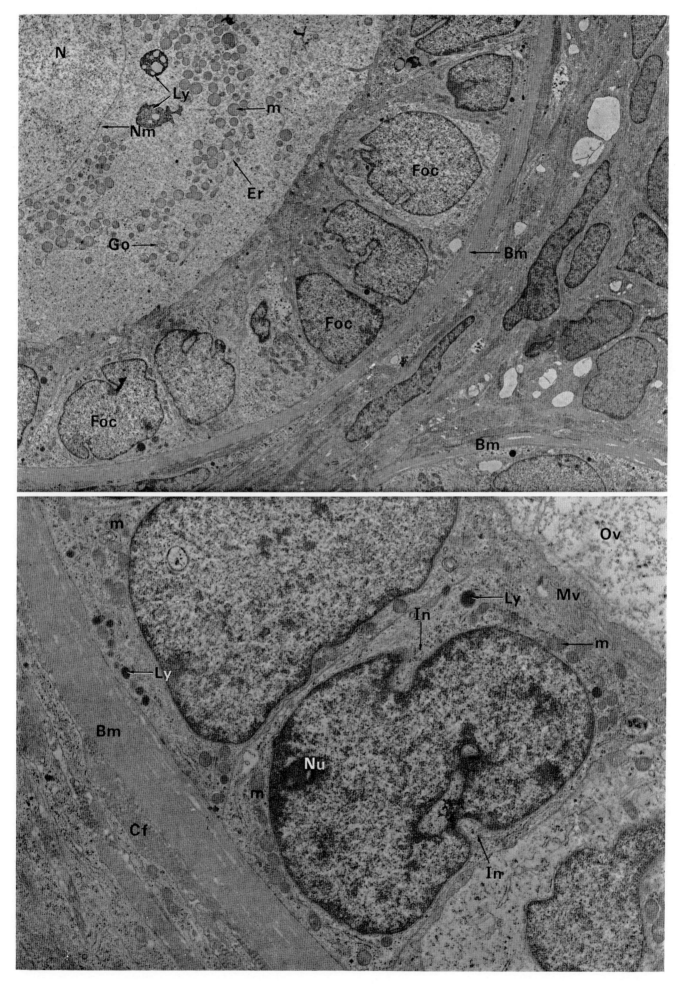

215

Annulate lamellae seen in a primary oocyte (Top)

In the oocyte are frequently seen annulate lamellae, clusters of parallel cisterns of smooth-surfaced membrane. They are perforated by numerous pores of about 700Å in diameter. These pores resemble those of the nuclear envelope and it is thought that the annulate lamellae may originate from the latter. Many authors regard the annulate lamellae as a specialized form of the endoplasmic reticulum, because the ends of individual cisterns often communicate with granular endoplasmic reticulum. However, their function is obscure at present.

This micrograph shows a portion of a primary oocyte containing annulate lamellae. Round mitochondria with a few cristae (m), strands of granular endoplasmic reticulum (Er) and a part of the nucleus (N) limited by a nuclear envelope (Nm) are also seen. Note the connection between cisterns of the annulate lamellae and those of the granular endoplasmic reticulum (arrows).

Developing zona pellucida of the oocyte (Bottom)

In the follicle covered by layers of follicle epithelial cells, the oocyte is surrounded by the zona pellucida, a specialized layer of polysaccharide-rich substance. This layer is, in light microscopy, clear and refractile and deeply stains in various dyes.

In this picture a peripheral portion of an oocyte, developing zona pellucida (*) and portions of the surrounding follicle epithelial cells (Foc) are shown. The zona pellucida consists of fine granular substance of moderate electron opacity. Microvillous structures (Mv) project into this layer from both oocyte and follicular cells.

Er : Granular endoplasmic reticulum.
Go : Golgi complex.
m : Mitochondrion.
N : Nucleus.
Nm : Nuclear membrane.

Top and Bottom : Material and method are the same as those of the photographs on page 215. Top : ×25,000. Bottom : ×17,000.

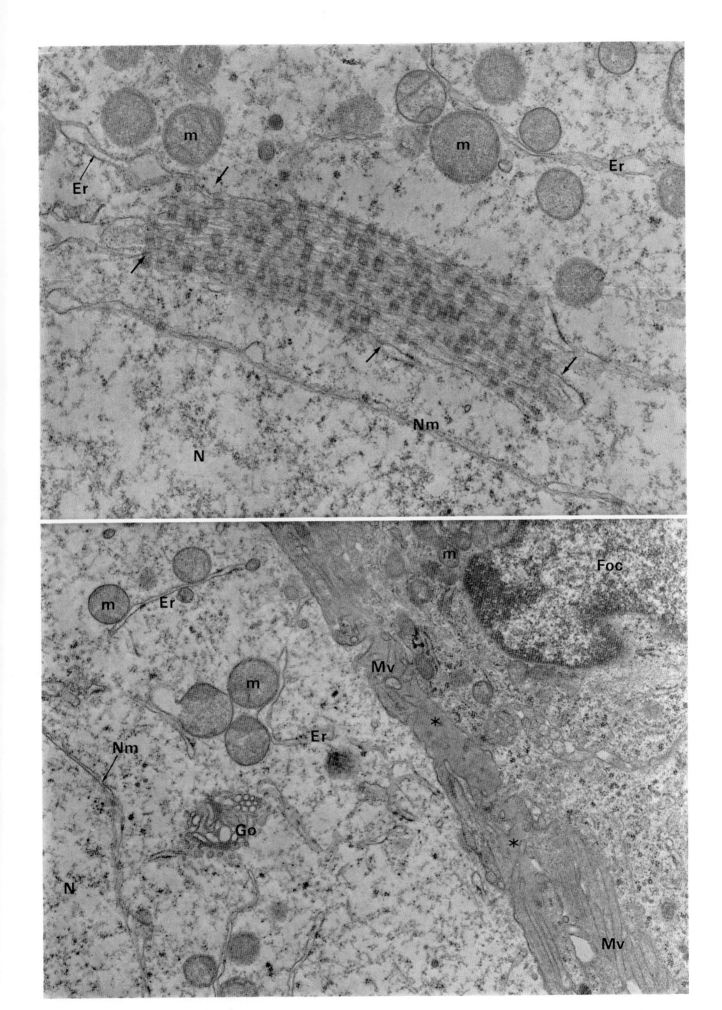

Granulosa lutein cell in the corpus luteum

The corpus luteum is an endocrine organ which secretes progesterone, a steroid hormone. It is formed from the wall of the ruptured ovarian follicle. Following ovulation, follicle epithelial cells increase in size and, at the same time, lipid droplets and yellow pigments begin to appear in their cytoplasm. These cells occupy the main part of the corpus luteum and are called granulosa lutein cells.

Under the electron microscope, the cytoplasm of the granulosa lutein cell is generally characterized by an abundance of tortuous, tubular, agranular endoplasmic reticulum, and by the occurrence of mitochondria with dense matrices and both tubular and lamellar cristae, and of numerous lipid droplets. These morphological features are common to such steroid-producing cells as adrenal cortical cells and the testicular interstitial cells. The yellow pigments seen in light microscopy correspond to the lysosomes in electron microscopy.

This electron micrograph shows portions of granulosa lutein cells seen in the corpus luteum twenty-five days after the beginning of the last menstruation. The cell surface is relatively smooth and closely apposed to that of the adjacent cells. In the upper left corner of this picture is a connective tissue which is separated from the lutein cells by a basal lamina (Bl). The nuclcolus (Nu) is large and prominent. In the cytoplasm, there are abundant profiles of mitochondria (m), a Golgi complex (Go), lipid droplets (Ld), large numbers of scattered ribosomes, granular (Er) and agranular endoplasmic reticulum (Ser), lysosomes (Ly) and bundles of cytoplasmic filaments (f).

Material and method are the same as those of the photographs on page 215. ×12,500.

REFERENCES:

ADAMS, E. C. and A. T. HERTIG: Studies on the human corpus luteum. I. Observations on the ultrastructure of development and regression of the luteal cells during the menstrual cycle. J. Cell Biol., *41*: 696–715, 1969.

ADAMS, E. C. and A. T. HERTIG: Studies on the human corpus luteum. II. Observations on the ultrastructure of luteal cells during pregnancy. J. Cell Biol., *41*: 716–735, 1969.

CRISP, T. M., D. A. DESSOUKY and F. R. DENYS: The fine structure of the human corpus luteum of early pregnancy and during the progestational phase of the menstrual cycle. Amer. J. Anat., *127*: 37–70, 1970.

GILLIM, S. W., A. K. CHRISTENSEN and C. E. McLENNAN: Fine structure of the human menstrual corpus luteum at its stage of maximum secretory activity. Amer. J. Anat., *126*: 409–428, 1969.

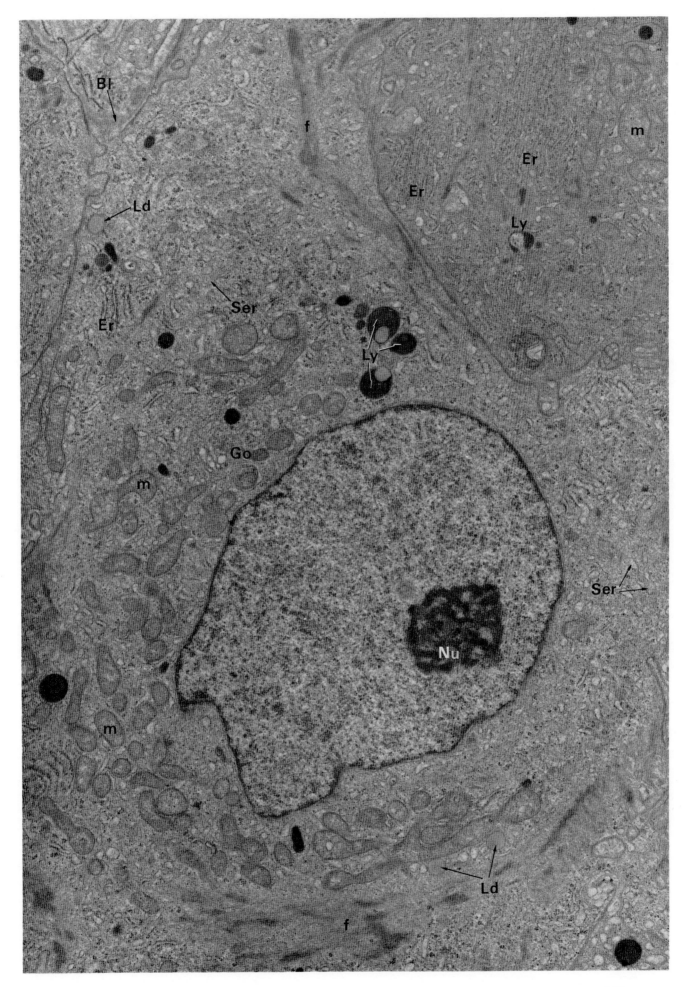

Epithelium of the endometrial gland (Top)

The surface and glandular epithelia as well as the connective tissue cells of the endometrium vary cyclically month by month in their structure.

This micrograph shows a portion of an endometrial gland in the proliferative phase. The epithelium is composed of two types of cells. One of these is a columnar cell with a small number of microvilli (Mv) on the luminal surface. The lateral surfaces are relatively smooth and the basal surface rests on the undulating basal lamina (Bl). The nucleus (N) with a prominent nucleolus (Nu) is elongated in shape, with its axis oriented in the long axis of the cell. The cytoplasm contains a few organelles such as mitochondria (m), strands of endoplasmic reticulum, lysosomes (Ly) and a poorly-developed Golgi complex. Epithelial cells of the second type are few in number and ciliated (Cil). They are scattered among columnar non-ciliated cells and have abundant mitochondria in the supranuclear region.

Lamina propria of the endometrium (Bottom)

The lamina propria of the endometrium consists of loose connective tissue containing characteristic stromal cells which are thought to be specially differentiated fibroblasts.

In this micrograph three profiles of stromal cells (Fb) are seen. The nuclei are large with prominent nucleoli (Nu). The cytoplasm contains abundant profiles of granular endoplasmic reticulum, mitochondria (m), lysosomes (Ly) and lipid droplets (Ld). The blood capillary (Cap) shown in the right side of this picture is lined by an endothelium surrounded by a thin basal lamina (Bl). Fine granular substances of low electron opacity are scattered between stromal cells.

Top and Bottom: Surgically-obtained uterus of a 32-year-old female with carcinoma colli (14 days after the beginning of the last menstruation). Phosphate-buffered 2.5% glutaraldehyde fixation followed by 1.0% osmium tetroxide post-fixation. Uranyl acetate and lead tartarate staining. Top: ×5,000. Bottom: ×4,000.

REFERENCES:

Cavazos, F., J. A. Green, D. G. Hall and F. V. Lucas: The microtubular system in the cytoplasm of the human endometrial glandular cell during the menstrual cycle. Amer. J. Obstet. Gynecol., *94*: 824–831, 1966.

Nilsson, O.: Correlation of structure to function of the luminal cell surface in the uterine epithelium of mouse and man. Z. Zellforsch., *56*: 803–808, 1962.

Nilsson, O.: Electron microscopy of the glandular epithelium in the human uterus. I. Follicular phase. J. Ultrastr. Res., *6*: 413–421, 1962.

Nilsson, O.: Electron microscopy of the glandular epithelium in the human uterus. II. Early and late luteal phase. J. Ultrastr. Res., *6*: 422–431, 1962.

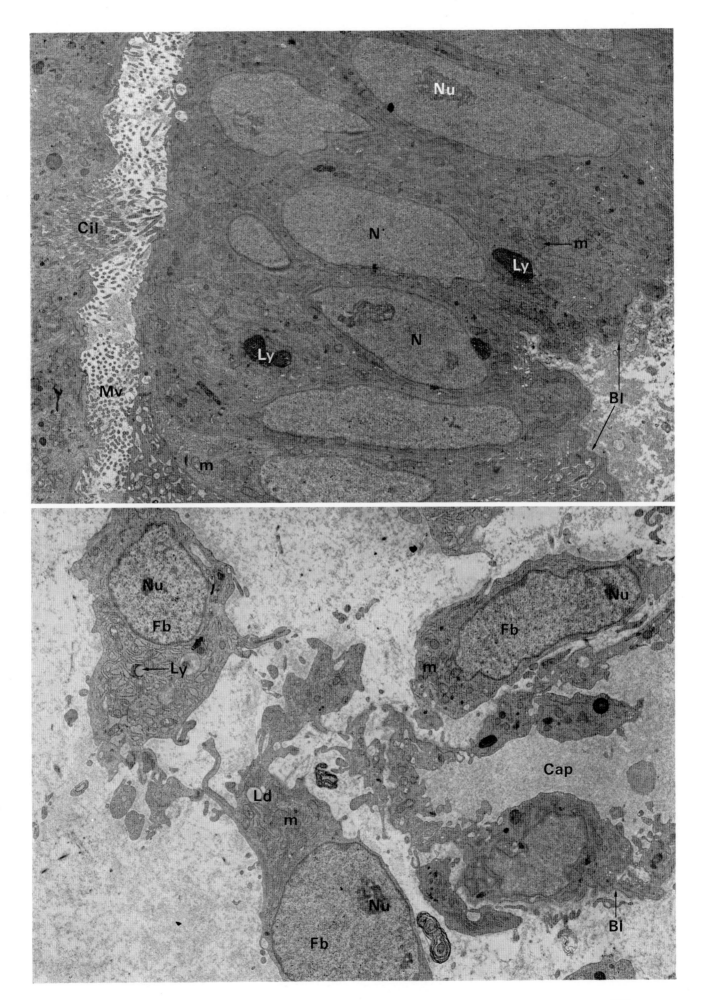

Coiled artery of the endometrium

The coiled arteries supply blood to the inner portion of the endometrium. By their constriction, the functional layer of the endometrium is cut off from the blood supply, causing its destruction. After the destroyed material has been shed, the arteries relax and the endometrium rebuilds itself from the basal layer.

These pictures show the coiled arteries in the proliferative stage of the endometrium. The endothelial cells show an elongated shape in a longitudinal section (Top) and a cuboidal one in a cross section (Bottom). Cell organelles such as granular endoplasmic reticulum, Golgi complex and mitochondrion, are well developed in comparison with other arteries of the same caliber. Smooth muscle fibers surrounding the endothelial cells contain abundant cell organelles. Myofilaments are usually few in number and are located in the peripheral portion of the cytoplasm.

Alu : Arterial lumen.
Bl : Basal lamina.
Ed : Endothelial cell.
Sm : Smooth muscle fiber.

Top and Bottom: Endometrium of a 28-year-old female (proliferative phase). Cacodylate-buffered 3.0% glutaraldehyde fixation followed by 2.0% osmium tetroxide post-fixation. Uranyl acetate and lead tartarate staining. Top and Bottom: ×4,500.

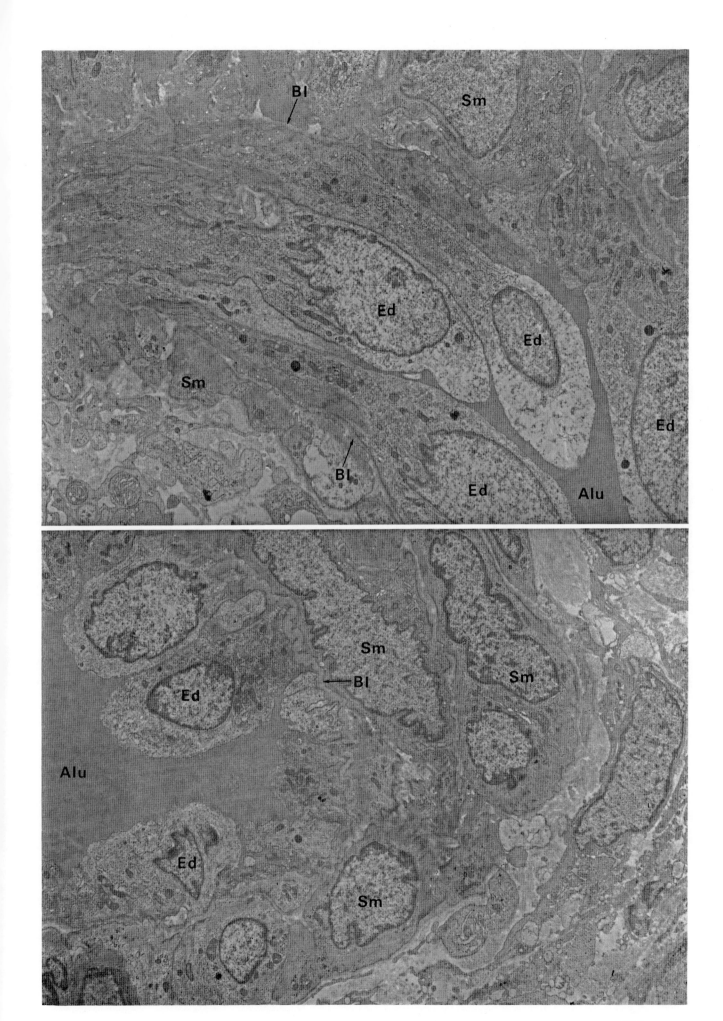

223

Chorionic villus

The placenta has two functions: first, it is the organ through which the fetus absorbs the nutriments from the maternal blood and excretes waste products into it, and second, it secretes hormones such as estrogen, progesterone and chorionic gonadotrophin. This organ consists of two parts, one of maternal origin and the other of fetal origin. The maternal portion is called decidua basalis and contains enlarged endometrial stromal cells known as decidual cells. The fetal portion is composed of the chorionic plate and the chorionic villi. The latter are bathed in the maternal blood that flows slowly through the intervillous space.

The chorionic villus is covered by a layer of syncytial trophoblasts and, until approximately the tenth week of pregnancy, by a layer of cytotrophoblasts or Langhans cells. The latter gradually disappear and, at child-birth, only isolated clumps of them remain. The fetal circulation is completely separated from the maternal one by a continuous layer of syncytial trophoblasts, a discontinuous layer of cytotrophoblast, a basal lamina lining both of them, a fetal connective tissue of gelatinous nature and a fetal capillary wall. These elements comprise the so-called placental barrier which permits the exchange of substances between the mother and the fetus.

Concerning the cellular origin of the placental hormones, it is probable that the syncytial trophoblasts secrete steroid hormones, estrogen and progesterone, whereas the cytotrophoblasts produce a proteinic hormone, chorionic gonadotrophin.

This micrograph shows a portion of a wall of a chorionic villus. Numerous microvilli (Mv) project from the surface of the syncytial trophoblast (Str) into the intervillous space (Ivs). The cytoplasm of the syncytial trophoblasts looks darker than that of the cytotrophoblasts (Lac). The core of the chorionic villus contains profiles of mesenchymal cells (Mec). A portion of a capillary is seen in the upper left corner (Ed).

Details of the small area enclosed in the box will be shown in the next picture.

Bl: Basal lamina.
Ld: Lipid droplet.
Mem: Mesenchymal matrix.

Placenta of a 7-week fetus. Phosphate-buffered 2.5% glutaraldehyde fixation followed by 1.0% osmium tetroxide post-fixation. Uranyl acetate and lead tartarate staining. ×5,500.

REFERENCES:

Boyd, J. D. and W. J. Hamilton: The human placenta. Heffer, Cambridge, 1970.

Björkman, N.: An atlas of placental fine structure. Baillière, London, 1970.

Rhodin, J. A. G. and J. Terzakis: The ultrastructure of the human full-term placenta. J. Ultrastr. Res., *6*: 88–106, 1962.

Terzakis, J. A.: The ultrastructure of normal human first trimester placenta. J. Ultrastr. Res., *9*: 268–284, 1963.

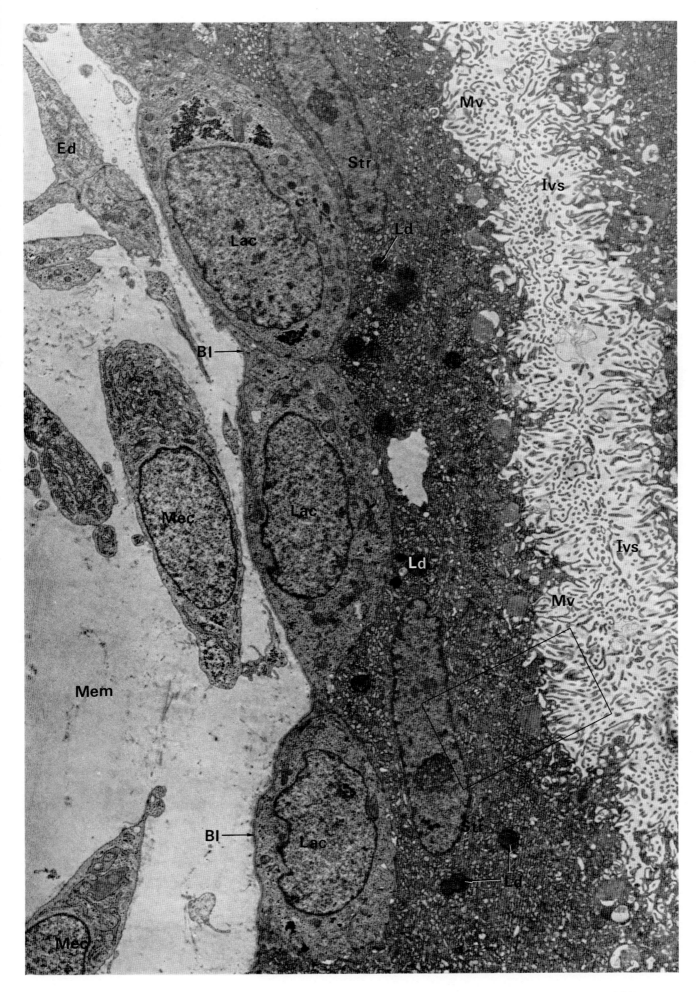

225

PLACENTA

Syncytial trophoblast (Top)

The name, syncytial trophoblast, is only historical because it is now evident that this kind of multinuclear cell is the product of repeated nuclear divisions and not of cell fusions.

This picture is an enlargement of the small area enclosed in the box in the picture on page 225. The cytoplasm of the syncytial trophoblast contains small mitochondria (m), a Golgi complex (Go) and abundant profiles of granular endoplasmic reticulum (Er). Cisterns of smooth-surfaced endoplasmic reticulum (Sr) contain an amorphous material of moderate electron density. They are thought to play a leading role in the production of estrogen and progesterone. Free ribosomes, microtubules and glycogen particles are scattered between other cell organelles. On the surface of the cell, there are many infoldings of plasma membrane (arrows), suggesting the pinocytotic activity of the cell. A large vacuole (Va) containing a fine granular material is seen immediately beneath the surface. A portion of the nucleus (N) is on the left side of this picture.

Cytotrophoblast and fetal capillary (Bottom)

Cytotrophoblasts or Langhans cells (Lac) of the chorionic villus are thought to be the site of production of a proteinic hormone, chorionic gonadotrophin. They are located between the syncytial trophoblast (Str) and the basal lamina (Bl). Their nucleus (N) is large with a conspicuous nucleolus (Nu). The cytoplasm is lighter than that of the syncytial trophoblast and contains Golgi complexes (Go), scattered profiles of granular endoplasmic reticulum (Er), small mitochondria (m) and large clusters of glycogen particles (Gl).

The capillary shown in this picture is lined solely by endothelial cells (Ed). The erythroblast (Ery) in the lumen is nucleated and contains a Golgi complex and mitochondria in its dense cytoplasm.

j: Junction between endothelial cells.
Mem: Mesenchymal matrix.

Top and Bottom: Material and method are the same as those of the picture on page 225. Top: ×23,000. Bottom: ×8,500.

REFERENCES:

ASHLEY, C. A.: Study of the human placenta with the electron microscope. Arch. Pathol., *80*: 377–390, 1965.

DEMPSEY, E. W. and S. A. LUSE: Regional specializations in the syncytial trophoblast of early human placentas. J. Anat., *108*: 545–561, 1971.

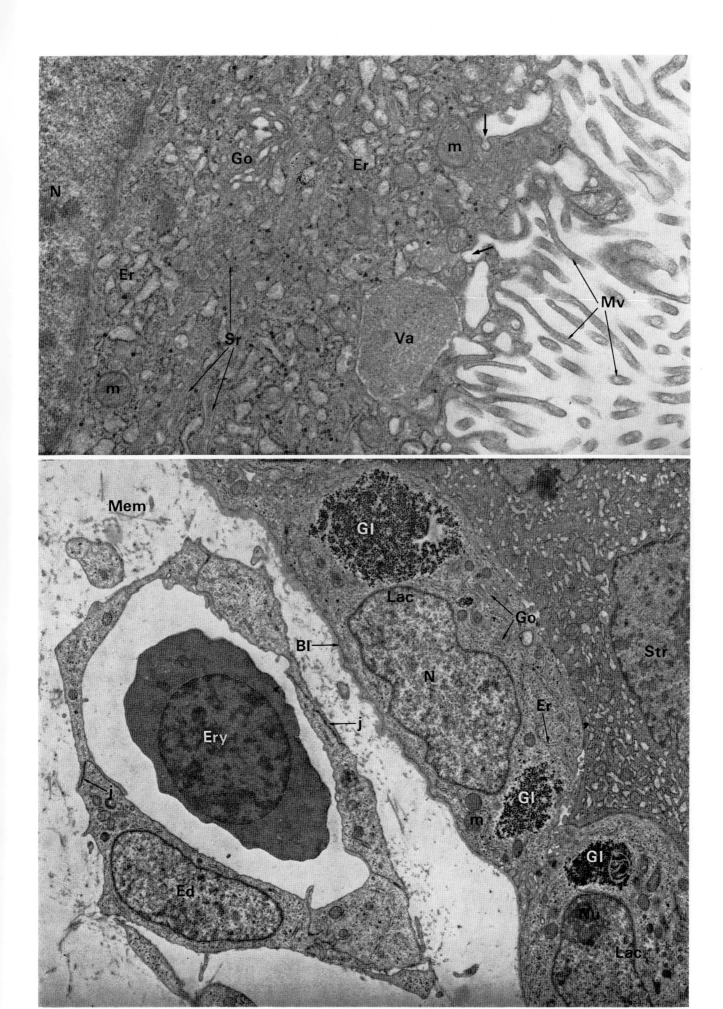

Pars distalis of the fetal adenohypophysis

The cells in the pars distalis (anterior lobe) are occasionally accumulated in a cluster to form a well-defined follicle as shown in this micrograph. A basal lamina (Bl) surrounds the cell cluster. Four types of cells are discernible in this micrograph: STH cell (STH or STH*), probable FSH cell (FSH), probable ACTH cell (ACTH) and undifferentiated cells (Uc).

The STH cell secretes growth hormone and corresponds to the typical acidophil in light microscopy. A detailed illustration of this type of cell is shown on page 231.

The FSH cell produces a follicle-stimulating hormone, one of the gonadotrophic hormones. This cell is thought to coincide with a kind of small-sized basophil in light microscopy. The granules of this cell are variable in electron density. In this micrograph the size of the granules ranges from 200 to 300 mμ in diameter.

The ACTH cell is believed to correspond to a type of large-sized basophil in light microscopy and produces the adrenocorticotrophic hormone. This cell projects several cytoplasmic processes from the peripheral surface. The granules of this cell are small in size, measuring 150 to 200 mμ in diameter.

The undifferentiated cell is poor in the development of cell organelles and contains no granules.

From the pituitary of a 7-month fetus (♂, 930 g). Phosphate-buffered 2.5% glutaraldehyde fixation followed by 1.0% osmium tetroxide post-fixation. Uranyl acetate and lead tartarate staining. ×5,400.

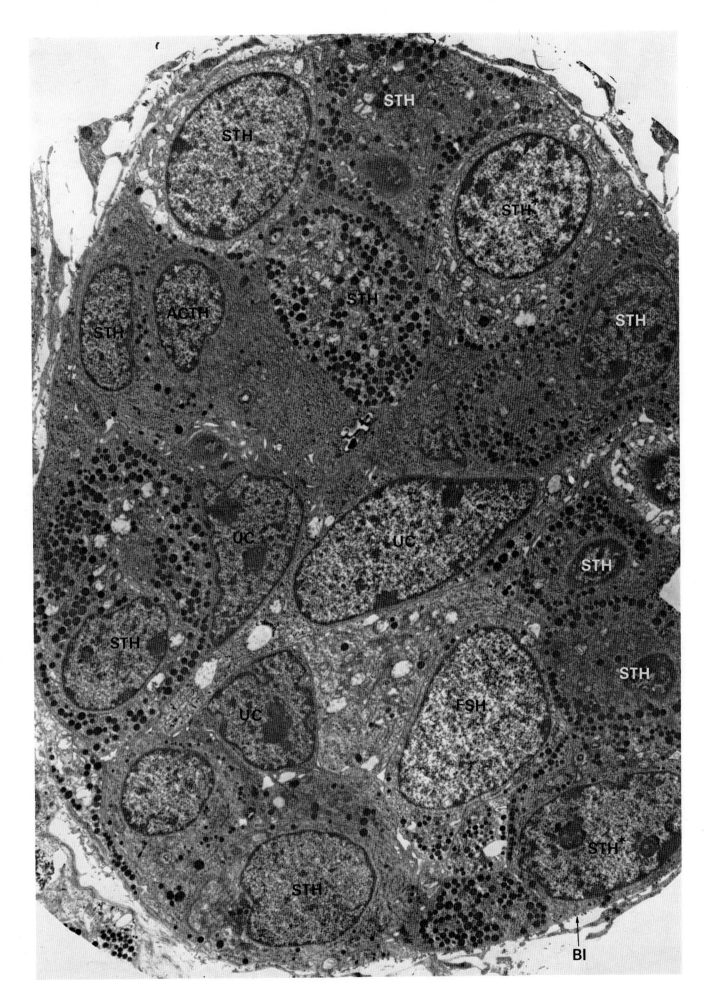

229

STH cell of the pars distalis

The STH cell is most frequently found in the anterior pituitary and is characterized by the presence of a large number of secretory granules which have a homogeneous internal texture with high electron density and measure 200 to 350 mμ in diameter. The granules are scattered throughout the cytoplasm as in the cell (STH$_1$) occupying the central portion of this micrograph, but they are occasionally gathered along the cell surface as shown in the cells marked by STH* in the micrograph on page 229. In the cell center, Golgi complexes (Go) and paired centrioles (c) are seen. Granular endoplasmic reticulum (Er) which consists of flattened cisterns is randomly oriented around the nucleus. It is often arranged in parallel as seen in the cell (STH$_2$) in the lower left corner. Mitochondria (m) are round or rod-like with numerous cristae.

    Gl: Glycogen particles.
    Nu: Nucleolus.
    Uc: Undifferentiated cell.

Material and method are the same as those of the picture on page 229.   ×11,500.

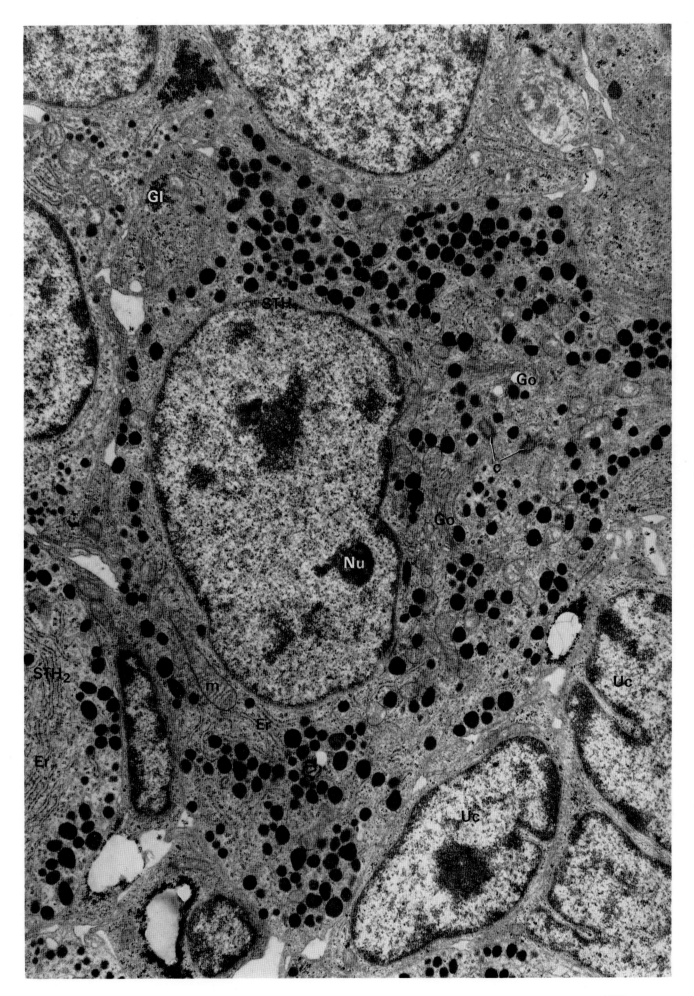

231

PITUITARY GLAND

Pituicyte in the fetal neurohypophysis

The neurohypophysis is the site of storage and release of oxytocin and vasopressin (anti-diuretic hormone). The tissue of this portion consists of pituicytes (Ptc) and non-myelinated nerve fibers (Ax).

The pituicytes, which are a kind of neuroglia, are intrinsic cells of the neurohypophysis. They have elongate nuclei (N). Golgi complexes (Go) showing lamellar sacs occur near the nuclei. Mitochondria (m) are small in size and mostly round in shape. Elements of granular endoplasmic reticulum (Er) are dispersed throughout the cyotplasm. Although lipid droplets are usually contained in the pituicyte of mammals, including adult man, none of them can be seen in this fetal material.

The numerous nerve fibers running among the pituicytes are originated from the neurosecretory cells in the hypothalamus. In the dilated cytoplasm of these fibers, a large number of dense granules (Sg) measuring 100 to 300 mμ in diameter are contained. These are the granules of neurosecretory substances formed in and transferred from the hypothalamus. An accumulation of small vesicles (v) is also contained within the cytoplasm of some axons. Vacuolar structures, which may correspond to the limiting membrane of the secretory granules after release of their content, are seen in other axons. Occasionally secretory granules, small vesicles and vacuolar structures are contained within one axon (arrow).

Material and method are the same as those of the picture on page 229. ×11,000.

232

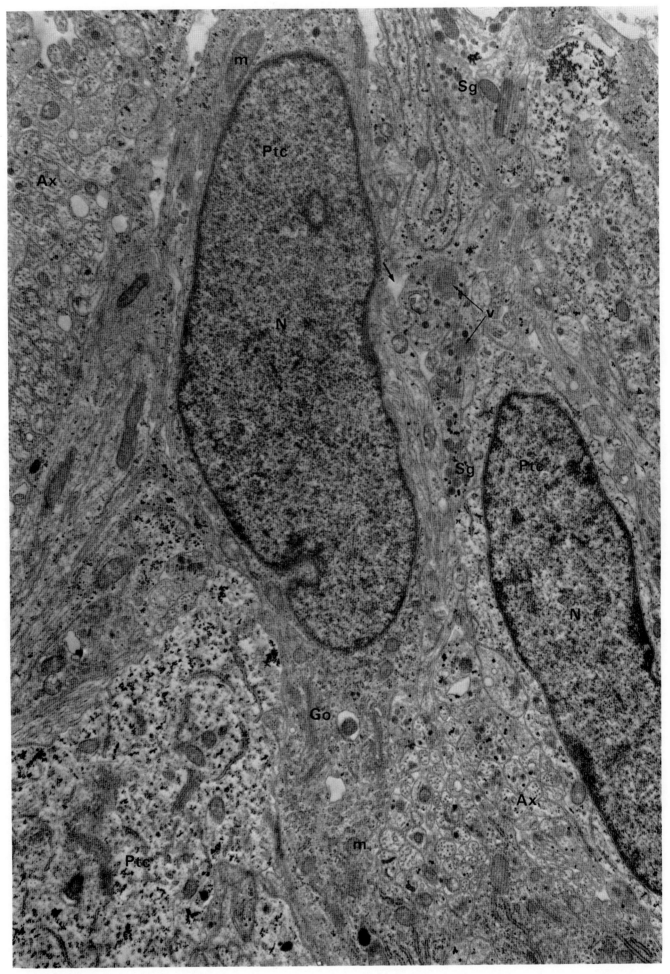

233

Thyroid follicle

The thyroid follicle is lined by a simple cuboidal epithelium.

The follicular lumen is filled with colloid containing thyroglobulin, a storage form of thyroid hormones synthesized in the follicular cells. This colloid is absorbed in the follicular cells, changed into active thyroid hormones (thyroxin and thyronin) after hydrolysis by their lysosomes and then released into the capillary (Cap). The follicular epithelial cells have a relatively large, spherical nucleus (N). The granular endoplasmic reticulum (Er) in the form of dilated cisterns is located throughout the cytoplasm. Numerous dense bodies (Db) occur in the supranuclear region. The follicles are surrounded by a thin basal lamina (Bl).

Nu : Nucleolus.
Co : Colloid.

Thyroid gland of a 7-month fetus (♂, 930 g). Phosphate-buffered 2.5% glutaraldehyde fixation followed by 1.3% osmium tetroxide post-fixation. Uranyl acetate and lead tartarate staining. ×5,000.

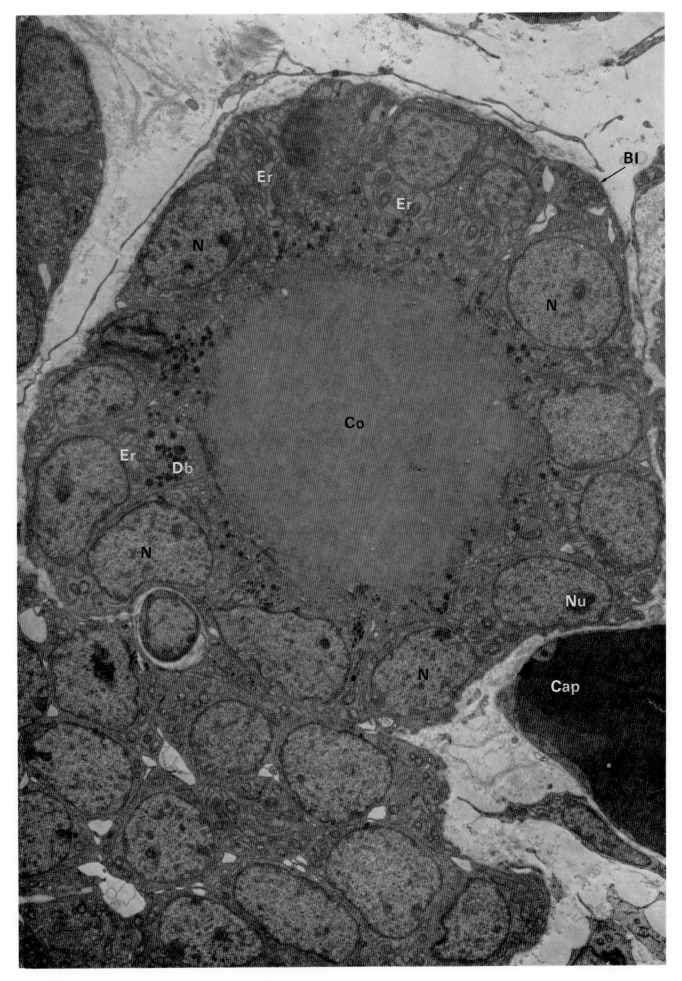

235

Apical portion of the follicular cell

The apical surface of follicular epithelial cells is provided with numerous microvilli (Mv). The lateral cell membranes are, near the lumen, tightly attached by a junctional complex (Jc). The supranuclear cytoplasm contains numbers of dense granules (Dg).

Co : Colloid
Er : Granular endoplasmic reticulum.
Go : Golgi complex.
m : Mitochondrion.
Nu : Nucleolus.

Material and method are the same as those of the picture on page 235.   ×28,000.

REFERENCE:

KLINCK, G. H., J. E. OERTEL and T. WINSHIP: Ultrastructure of normal human thyroid. Lab. Invest., *22:* 2-22, 1970.

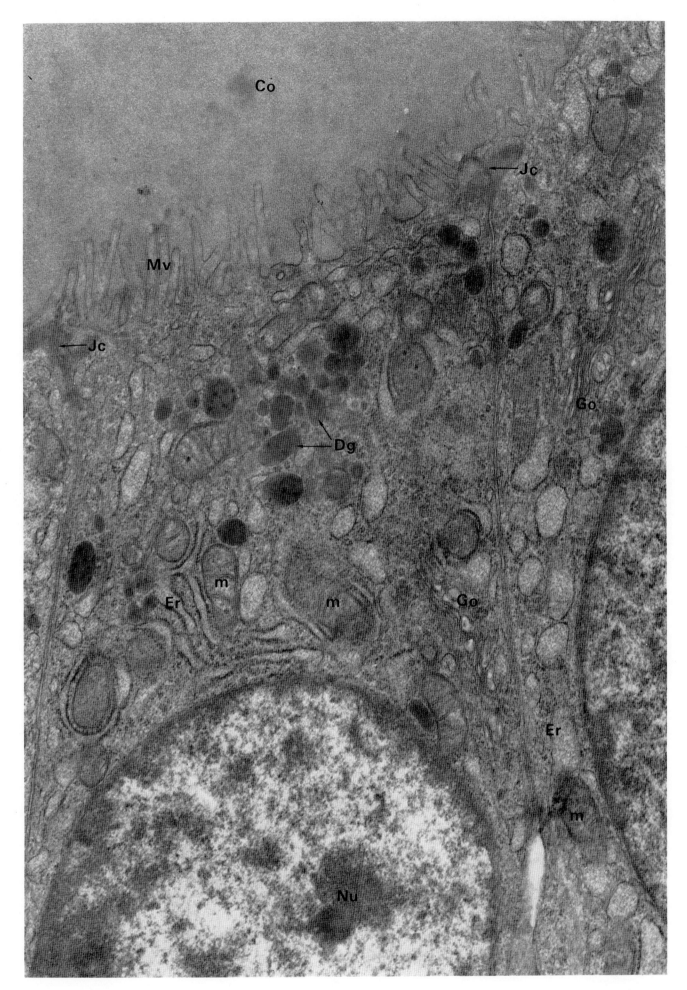

237

Cell of the inner layer of the fetal adrenal cortex

In early fetal life, the adrenal cortex arises from the mesoderm near the cephalic pole of the mesonephros. From the third month of pregnancy until shortly after birth, the adrenal cortex consists of a narrow outer zone of small cells and an inner zone consisting of cords of large cells lying between blood capillaries. From the outer zone develops the adult cortex, while the inner zone is destined to undergo involution within two to four weeks of birth, though it may already be active in steroid-secretion in the fetal life.

This micrograph shows the fine structure of the cell of the inner zone of the fetal adrenal cortex. The nucleus is ovoid in shape, with a prominent nucleolus (Nu). Chromation is located in the periphery of the nucleus. The most characteristic feature of the cytoplasm is probably the presence of abundant profiles of agranular endoplasmic reticulum (Ser). In the adrenal cortical cell, the agranular endoplasmic reticulum forms a three-dimensional network of interconnected tubules. Mitochondria (m) are variable in size and characterized by dense matrices and tubular or vesicular cristae. A dense material (arrows) is frequently present in the mitochondrial matrices, but there are no intramitochondrial granules. Flattened cisterns of granular endoplasmic reticulum (Er) are assembled in a parallel arrangement in several portions of the cytoplasm. A small number of lipid droplets (Ld) is also seen between the cell organelles mentioned above.

Adrenal cortex of a 6-month fetus (♀, 800 g). Phosphate-buffered glutaraldehyde fixation followed by 1.0% osmium tetroxide post-fixation. Uranyl acetate and lead tartarate staining. ×10,000.

REFERENCES:

CARR, I.: The ultrastructure of the human adrenal cortex before and after stimulation with ACTH. J. Pathol. Bacteriol., *81*: 101–106, 1961.

LONG, J. A. and A. L. JONES: Observations on the fine structure of the adrenal cortex of man. Lab. Invest., *17*: 355–370, 1967.

McNUTT, N. S. and A. L. JONES: Observations on the ultrastructure of cytodifferentiation in the human fetal adrenal cortex. Lab. Invest., *22*: 513–527, 1970.

ROSS, M. H., G. D. PAPPAS, J. T. LANMAN and J. LIND: Electron microscope observations on the endoplasmic reticulum in the human fetal adrenal. J. biophysic. biochem. Cytol., *4*: 659–662, 1958.

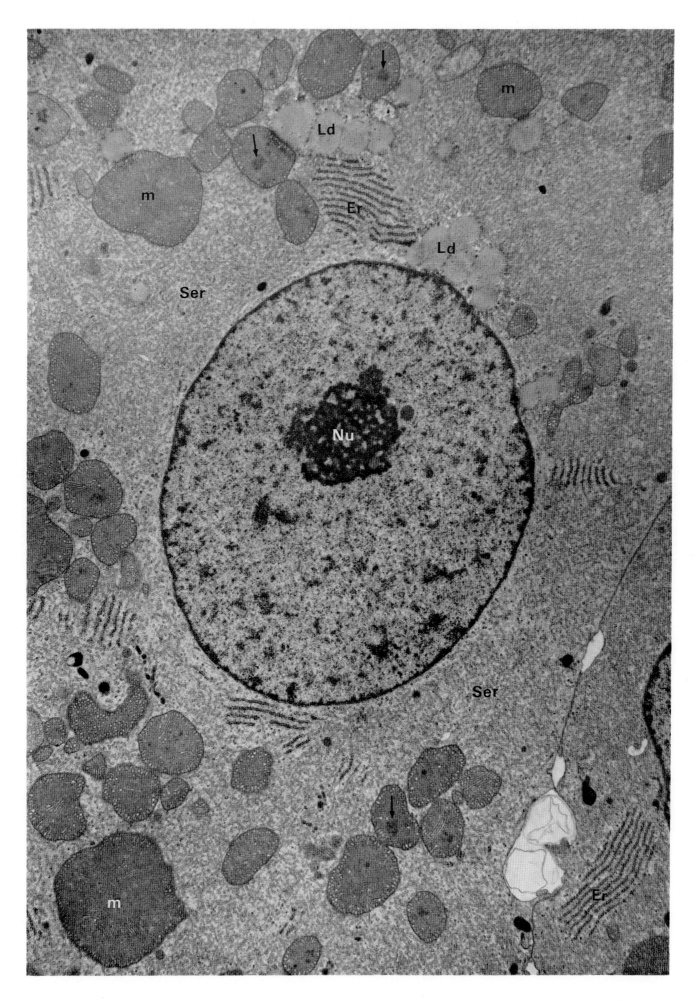

Cell of the adrenal cortical adenoma associated with Cushing's syndrome

The adrenal cortex in the adult consists of three ill-defined layers: a thin outer zone, zona glomerulosa; a thick middle zone, zona fasciculata; and an inner zone, zona reticularis. Cells of the zona glomerulosa elaborate mineralocorticoids, hormones which control electrolytes and water balance. Cells of the zona fasciculata are known to secrete glucocorticoids, hormones which participate in carbohydrate metabolism. Cells of the zona reticularis produce both female and male sex hormones.

This micrograph shows a portion of an adenoma cell of a patient suffering from Cushing's syndrome. The endocrine disturbances in this patient (hypertension, moon face, obesity of trunk and so forth), which are a manifestation of hyperglucocorticoidism, suggest that the adenoma of this patient arose from the zona fasciculata.

In the lower left corner is a portion of the nucleus (N) which is separated from the cytoplasm by a nuclear envelope perforated by nuclear pores. There are prominent cisterns of granular endoplasmic reticulum (Er) on the right side of this picture. They are assembled in stacks of more than twenty parallel units. The cytoplasm between the nucleus and parallel-arranged cisterns of granular endoplasmic reticulum is mostly filled with a network of tubular, agranular endoplasmic reticulum (Ser). Continuity between agranular and granular endoplasmic reticulum is occasionally found (arrows). Mitochondria (m) and several profiles of lysosomes (Ly) are also seen. The cell surface provided with microvilli (Mv) is in the upper right corner.

Surgically-removed adrenal cortical adenoma of a 12-year-old female with Cushing's syndrome. Cacodylate-buffered 4.0% glutaraldehyde fixation followed by 2.0% osmium tetroxide post-fixation. Uranyl acetate and lead tartarate staining. ×32,000. (Photograph courtesy of Dr. K. KANO)

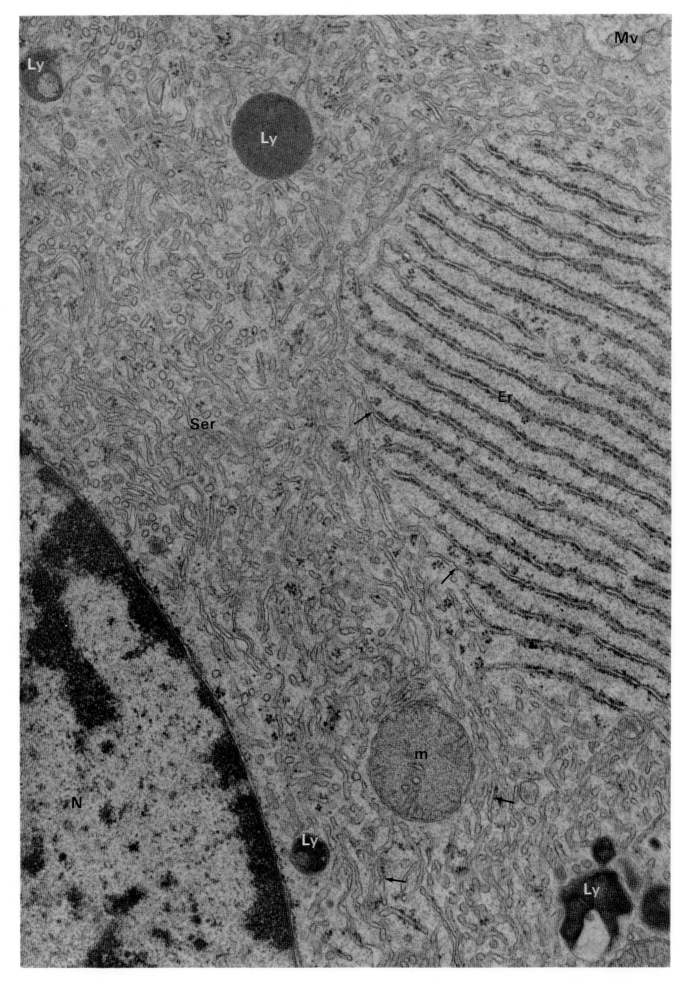

241

Epidermis

The human epidermis is a keratinized, stratified squamous epithelium in which two distinct systems of cells live together. The first is the keratinocytes, comprising most of the epidermis. The second is the epidermal dendritic cells in which two types of cells, the melanocytes and Langerhans cells, are known.

The superficial keratinized cells are continually exfoliated from the body surface as dirt and are constantly renewed from the element of the deeper layer. Mitotic activity is confined to the deepest portion of the epidermis and the newly-formed cells move upward. As they are displaced to higher levels, they become flattened and undergo a process of keratinization. When most of the cytoplasm is replaced by keratin, the cells die, resulting in the formation of dry, tough scales.

In the abdominal epidermis shown in this picture, four layers are distinguished. They are stratum basale, stratum spinosum, stratum granulosum and stratum corneum. The stratum basale consists of a single layer of columnar keratinocytes containing an oval nucleus with a distinct nucleolus. The stratum spinosum consists of two to three layers of polyhedral keratinocytes with a round nucleus and a conspicuous nucleolus. In both layers, the surface of the keratinocytes is covered with numerous short projections which meet with similar projections of adjacent cells, resulting in the formation of the so-called intercellular bridges (arrows). The cytoplasm contains dense tonofibrile bundles. These are randomly oriented, but in the stratum spinosum, they tend to aggregate at the periphery of the cells and terminate in desmosomes. In the keratinocytes of the stratum basale, numerous melanin granules are scattered among the bundles of tonofibrils. The keratinocytes of the stratum granulosum are flattened and contain a flattened nucleus and numerous keratohyalin granules (Kg) in the cytoplasm. In the keratinocytes of the stratum corncum almost all cell organelles and nuclei have disappeared. The cytoplasm is filled with keratin and appears homogeneous and dense. Most of the stratum corneum is lost from this picture.

A Langerhans cell (Lc) is seen in the stratum spinosum. Some processes of melanocytes (Mc) are intercalated between the keratinocytes of the stratum basale.

Der: Dermis.

Abdominal skin of a 72-year-old male with rectal cancer. Obtained during surgical operation. Phosphate-buffered 2.5% glutaraldehyde fixation followed by post-fixation with 2.0% osmium tetroxide solution. Uranyl acetate and lead tartarate staining. ×4,200.

REFERENCES:

BREATHNACH, A. S.: An atlas of the ultrastructure of human skin. Development, differentiation, and post-natal features. Churchill, London, 1971.

ZELICKSON, A. S. (ed.): Ultrastructure of normal and abnormal skin. Lea & Febiger, Philadelphia, 1967.

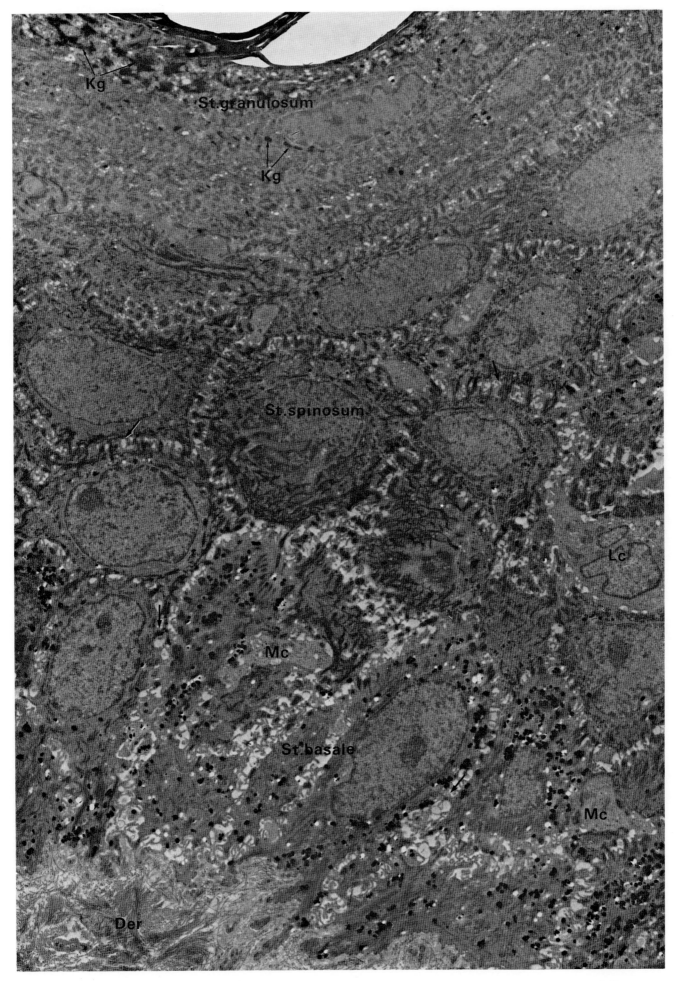

243

Keratinocyte in the stratum basale (Top)

Apical portions of keratinocytes of the stratum basale are shown. Their surface is highly irregular in outline and provided with a large number of cytoplasmic extensions meeting at desmosomes (d). The cytoplasm contains abundant tonofilaments (f), some of which converge on the desmosome. The cytoplasm also contains numerous free ribosomes, a few profiles of granular endoplasmic reticulum, a Golgi complex (Go), some mitochondria (m) and dense particles of melanin (Mp). The melanin particles are not elaborated by the keratinocyte itself, but they have been produced by the melanocyte and released into intercellular space to be engulfed and stored by the keratinocyte.

     Is :   Intercellular space.
     N :   Nucleus.

Abdominal skin of a 72-year-old male with rectal cancer. Obtained by operation. Phosphate-buffered 2.5% glutaraldehyde fixation followed by post-fixation with 2.0% osmium tetroxide solution. Uranyl acetate and lead citrate staining. ×16,000. (Photograph courtesy of Dr. H. OZAWA)

Dermo-epidermal junction (Bottom)

The junction between the epithelial and connective tissue components of the skin, whose nature and changes are important items of study from the viewpoint of investigative and clinical dermatology, is characterized by an occurrence of half desmosomes or hemi-desmosomes represented by spotty concentrations of cellular and extracellular materials on this junction.

In this picture a large area of the keratinocyte is occupied by randomly oriented tonofilaments (f), some of which converge on the hemi-desmosomes resting on the basal lamina (Bl). Between tonofilaments, free ribosomes (r) are dispersed.

     Der :   Dermis
     Hd :   Hemi-desmosome.
     t :   Microtubule.

Material and method are the same as those of the top picture. ×62,000. (Photograph courtesy of Dr. H. OZAWA)

REFERENCES:

BRODY, I.: The ultrastructure of the tonofibrils in the keratinization process of normal human epidermis. J. Ultrastr. Res., *4*: 264–297, 1960.

CHARLES, A. and F. G. SMIDDY: The tonofibrils of the human epidermis. J. Invest. Dermatol., *29*: 327–338, 1957.

PEARSON, R. W. and B. SPARGO: Electron microscope studies on dermal-epidermal separation in human skin. J. Invest. Dermatol., *36*: 213–224, 1961.

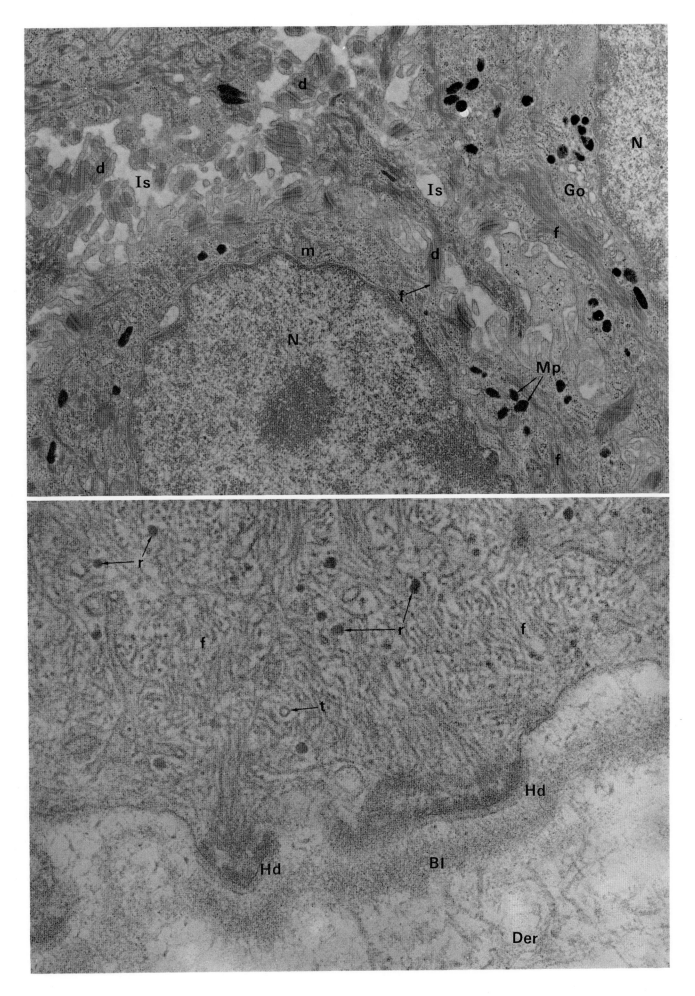

Junction between keratinocytes in the stratum spinosum

The keratinocyte in the stratum spinosum is called prickle cell because it possesses numerous spines on its surface. The spines of adjacent prickle cells are attached by numerous desmosomes and occasionally by tight junctions. Because two cell membranes at the junction can not be resolved by light microscopy, it was previously thought that adjacent prickle cells were joined by the intercellular bridges to communicate with one another. However, electron microscopy has shown that there is no protoplasmic continuity between adjacent prickle cells.

Top: Desmosomes and a tight junction (macula occludens) formed between five profiles of keratinocytes in the stratum spinosum of the epidermis.

Bottom: Desmosomes formed between two keratinocytes of the stratum spinosum of the epidermis. Three dense layers are noticed in the intercellular space, and two concentrations of apparently different dense materials are in the cytoplasm.

Is: Intercellular space.
Mv: Microvillus projecting into the intercellular space.
r: Free ribosome.
f: Tonofibrils inserting themselves into the desmosome.
Mo: Tight junction (macula occludens).
I, II, III, IV, V: Profiles of keratinocytes in the stratum spinosum.

Material and method are the same as those of the pictures on page 245. Top: ×87,000. Bottom: ×165,000. (Photographs courtesy of Dr. H. Ozawa)

REFERENCES:

Hibbs, R.G. and W.H. Clark: Electron microscope studies of the human epidermis. The cell boundaries and topography of the stratum malpighii. J. biophysic. biochem. Cytol., 6: 71–76, 1959.

Karrer, H.E.: Cell interconnections in normal human cervical epithelium. J. biophysic. biochem. Cytol., 7: 181–184, 1960.

Odland, G.F.: The fine structure of the interrelationship of cells in the human epidermis. J. biophysic. biochem. Cytol., 4: 529–538, 1958.

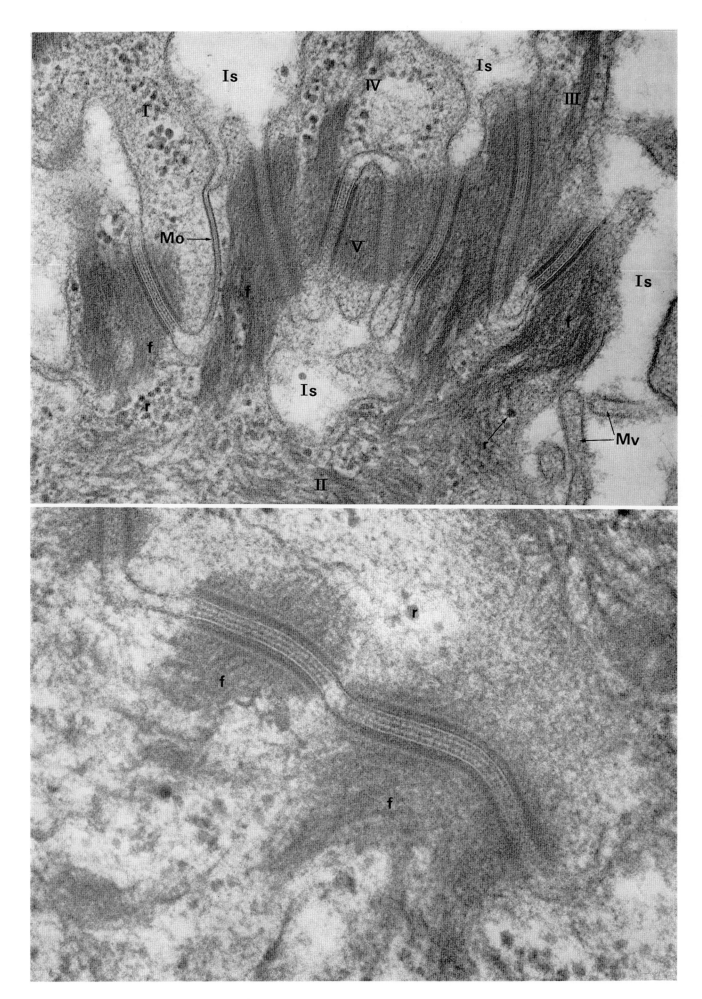

247

Langerhans cell

The Langerhans cell is a kind of dendritic cell of the epidermis which was found with the gold chloride method by P. Langerhans in 1868. It is located mainly in the stratum spinosum but sometimes occurs in the stratum basale. Although several authors consider it related to melanocytes, its real function remains obscure at present.

Top: A portion of the stratum spinosum of the epidermis.

Several keratinocytes and a Langerhans cell are shown. The surface of the keratinocyte is covered by numerous cytoplasmic processes which connect with similar processes of adjacent keratinocytes to form intercellular bridges. The cytoplasm of the keratinocyte contains, together with a few cell organelles, abundant bundles of tonofilaments.

The Langerhans cell has a nucleus (N) which is highly irregular in outline. Its cytoplasm contains a well-developed Golgi complex (Go) and oval mitochondria (m). The Langerhans cell does not form a desmosome against adjacent keratinocytes. The clear appearance of the cytoplasm of the Langerhans cell may be due to the lack of tonofilaments. Processes of the Langerhans cell (Pr) are intercalated between keratinocytes.

Bottom: A Golgi area of a Langerhans cell including Birbeck's granules (Bg).

The granules in Langerhans cells of the human epidermis were first described by BIRBECK and his co-workers (1961). In the ultrathin section, they appear like rod-shaped, membrane-limited granules with a central linear density at one end of the rod; some of them have a vesicular portion shaped like a tennis racket (arrows).

Although the function of the granules is not known as yet, it may be worthy of mention that they are found not only in Langerhans cells, but also in various cells of macrophage-like appearance in the lymphoid and connective tissues of the body.

Go: Golgi complex.
m: Mitochondrion.
N: Nucleus

Top and Bottom: Material and method are the same as those of the picture on page 243. Top: ×5,500. Bottom: ×39,000.

REFERENCES:

BELL, M.: Langerhans granules in fetal keratinocytes. J. Cell Biol., *41*: 914–918, 1969.

BIRBECK, M. S., A. S. BREATHNACH and J. D. EVERALL: An electron microscope study of basal melanocytes and high-level clear cells (Langerhans cells) in vitiligo. J. Invest. Dermatol., *37*: 51–64, 1961.

BREATHNACH, A. S.: The epidermal Langerhans cell. Brit. J. Dermatol., *80*: 688–689, 1968.

BREATHNACH, A. S.: The cell of Langerhans. Int. Rev. Cytol., *18*: 1–28, 1965.

KISTALA, U. and K. K. MUSTAKALLIO: Electron microscopic evidence of synthetic activity in Langerhans cells of human epidermis. Z. Zellforsch., *78*: 427–440, 1967.

SAGEBIEL, R. W. and T. H. REED: Serial reconstruction of the characteristic granule of the Langerhans cell. J. Cell Biol., *36*: 595–602, 1968.

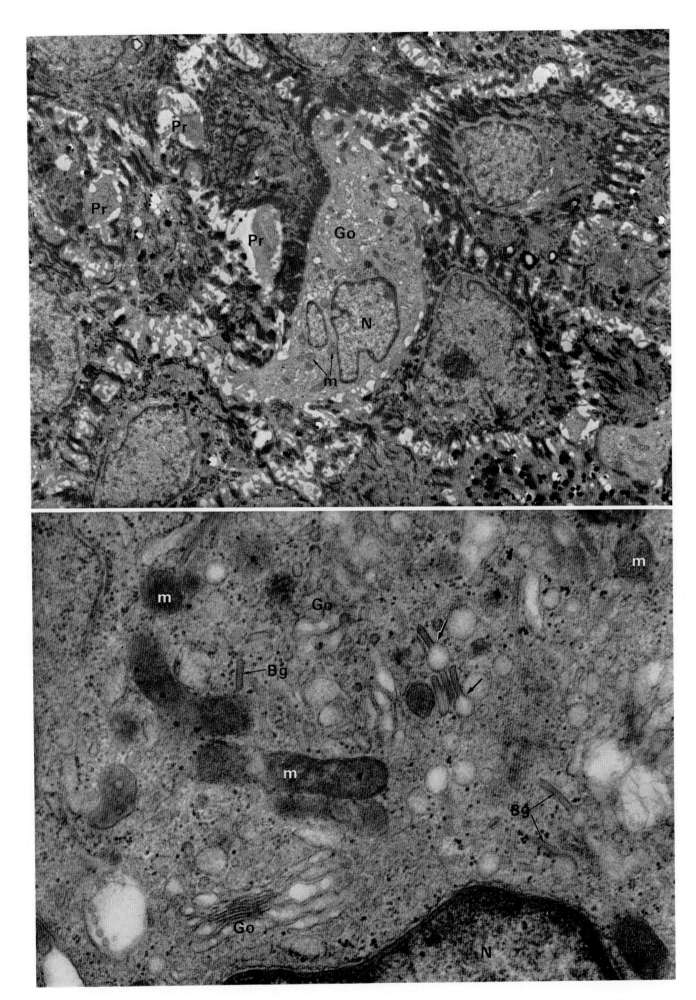

249

Melanocyte

The melanocyte, or melanin-producing cell, is a dendritic epidermal cell which has migrated from the neural crest and is usually located at the stratum basale. Its cytoplasm contains numerous melanosomes, specific granules of elongate forms, in which melanin is formed.

Top: This is an electron micrograph of the stratum basale of the human fetal epidermis showing a melanocyte (Mlc) and several developing keratinocytes (Krc).

The melanocyte is the only site of melanin production in the human epidermis. It is now accepted that the fully-formed melanosome is transferred from the melanocyte to the adjacent keratinocytes, though the exact mechanism of this transport remains obscure. Although in the adult human skin, numerous melanosomes are seen in the keratinocytes rather than in the melanocytes, the keratinocytes in the fetal epidermis do not contain melanosomes. The melanocyte is not attached by desmosomes to neighboring keratinocytes. Its cytoplasm appears lighter than that of the keratinocyte owing to the lack of tonofilaments.

Bl: Basal lamina separating the epidermis from the dermis.
d: Desmosome.
Is: Intercellular space.
m: Mitochondrion.
Ms: Melanosome.
f: Tonofilament.

From the scalp of a 6-month fetus (♀, 600 g). Phosphate-buffered 2.5% glutaraldehyde fixation followed by post-fixation with 1.3% osmium tetroxide solution. Stained with lead tartarate solution. ×11,500.

Bottom: Cross section of a process of melanocyte intercalated between two keratinocytes. Melanosomes (Ms) in various stages of development are seen. They are ovoid or rod-shaped bodies limited by a membrane sac. The mature melanosome contains dense amorphous material in its membrane sac; on the other hand, the younger ones are characterized by contents of striated appearance.

Is: Intercellular space.
Kg: Keratohyalin granule.
Mv: Microvilli projecting from the keratinocyte.
r: Free ribosome.
f: Tonofilament.

From the stratum basale of the abdominal epidermis of a 60-year-old male with rectal cancer. Obtained by surgical operation. Phosphate-buffered 2.5% glutaraldehyde fixation followed by post-fixation with 2.0% osmium tetroxide solution. Uranyl acetate and lead citrate staining. ×79,000. (Photograph courtesy of Dr. H. OZAWA)

REFERENCES:

CHARLES, A. and J. T. INGRAM: Electron microscope observations of the melanocytes of the human epidermis. J. biophysic. biochem. Cytol., *6*: 41–44, 1959.

CLARK, W. H. and R. G. HIBBS: Electron microscope studies of the human epidermis. The clear cell of Masson (dendritic cell or melanocyte). J. biophysic. biochem. Cytol., *4*: 679–684, 1958.

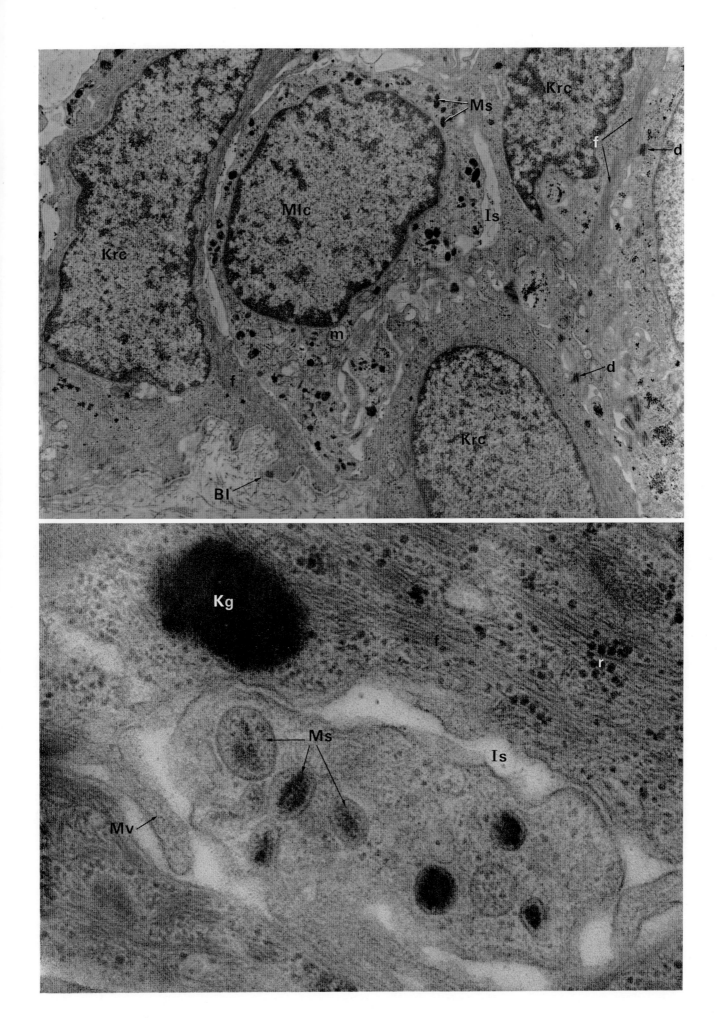

Junction between the stratum corneum and stratum granulosum (Top)

In the upper half of this picture, portions of two cornified cells are shown. In the space between them, an amorphous intercellular substance is seen (Ics). Dense structures (Ds) seen in the cornified cell are presumably remnants of either the nucleus or keratohyalin granules. Note "keratin pattern" in the cytoplasm of the cornified cell: The tonofibrils are embedded in the dense keratohyalin material so that they are viewed as a relatively electron lucent structure against a dark background. Note also the desmosome (d) between the granular cell and cornified cell. Half of the desmosome attached to the former appears typical, but the other half attached to the latter possesses no definite attachment plaque. The cytoplasm of the granular cell contains dense deposits of keratohyalin (Kg) on the tonofibrils.

Abdominal skin of a 59-year-old male with rectal cancer. Obtained by operation. Phosphate-buffered 2.5% glutaraldehyde followed by 2.0% osmium tetroxide post-fixation. Uranyl acetate and lead tartarate staining. ×64,000. (Photograph courtesy of Dr. H. Ozawa)

Odland body and desmosome in the stratum granulosum (Bottom)

The Odland body (Od) occurs in the cells of the stratum spinosum and stratum granulosum of the epidermis. It is an ovoid, membrane-bound granule of 100 to 300 mμ in diameter, containing a lamellar structure. It is said that the content of the Odland body covers the cell surface and serves to protect the epidermis from the keratinolytic agents. It has also been suggested that it is of lysosomal nature to facilitate the exfoliation of cornified squamous cells.

On the upper side of the cell surface, the cell membrane is invaginated to continue to the boundary of the Odland body (arrows). This figure suggests the emiocytotic discharge of the lamellar contents of the body.

Desmosomes (d) in the stratum granulosum have a much denser intercellular substance than those in the stratum spinosum. Tonofibrils (f) in the cytoplasm converge on the desmosomes.

Kg: Keratohyalin granule.

Material and method are the same as those of the top picture. ×138,000. (Photograph courtesy of Dr. H. Ozawa)

REFERENCE:

Wolff, K. und K. Holubar: Odland-Körper (membrane coating granules, Keratino-somen) als epidermale Lysosomen. Ein elektronenmikroskopischer Beitrag zur Verhornungsprozeß der Haut. Arch. klin. exp. Dermatol., *231*: 1–19, 1967.

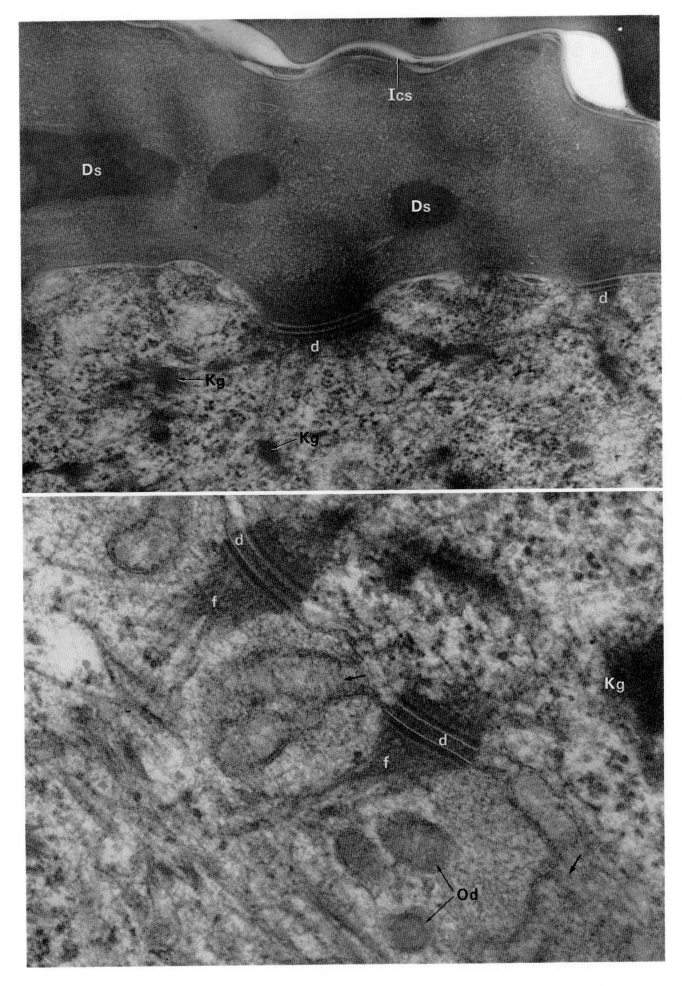

253

Hair follicle of the fetus

The hair follicle is the sheath which encloses the hair shaft and is derived from an epidermal invagination. Though usually composed of two layers, the outer and the inner root sheath, it varies in structure according to the depth from the skin surface.

Top : This micrograph shows a cross section of a hair follicle near the skin surface where it consists of only an outer root sheath. This sheath is a stratified squamous epithelium covered, as is the epidermis itself, with a keratinized layer, the stratum corneum (Corn). The subsequent single layer of the squamous cells containing keratohyalin granules (Kg) corresponds to the stratum granulosum (Gran), and the remaining layer of the stratified cells which contain a large amount of glycogen particles to the stratum germinativum (Germ). The hair shaft is not seen in this micrograph.

      Bl : Basal lamina.
      Cf : Collagenous fiber.
      N : Nucleus.

Bottom : This micrograph shows a cross section of a hair follicle at a level between the sebaceous gland orifice and the hair bulb. Both inner and outer root sheaths are seen here. The inner sheath consists of a keratinized epithelium of two layers : Huxley's and Henle's layers. The outer sheath is characterized by an abundance of glycogen particles. The outer surface of the follicle is outlined by a thin basal lamina (Bl) and surrounded by the connective tissue sheath containing thick collagenous fibers (Cf).

      Cu : Developing cuticle of inner root sheath.
      Fc : Fibrocyte.
      Hux : Huxley's layer, in which trichohyalin granules (Tr) are abundantly contained.
      Hen : Henle's layer.
      N : Nucleus.
      Ors : Outer root sheath.

Top and Bottom : Scalp of a 7-month fetus (♀, 600 g). Method for specimen preparation is the same as that of the picture on page 243. Top : ×3,500. Bottom : ×4,000.

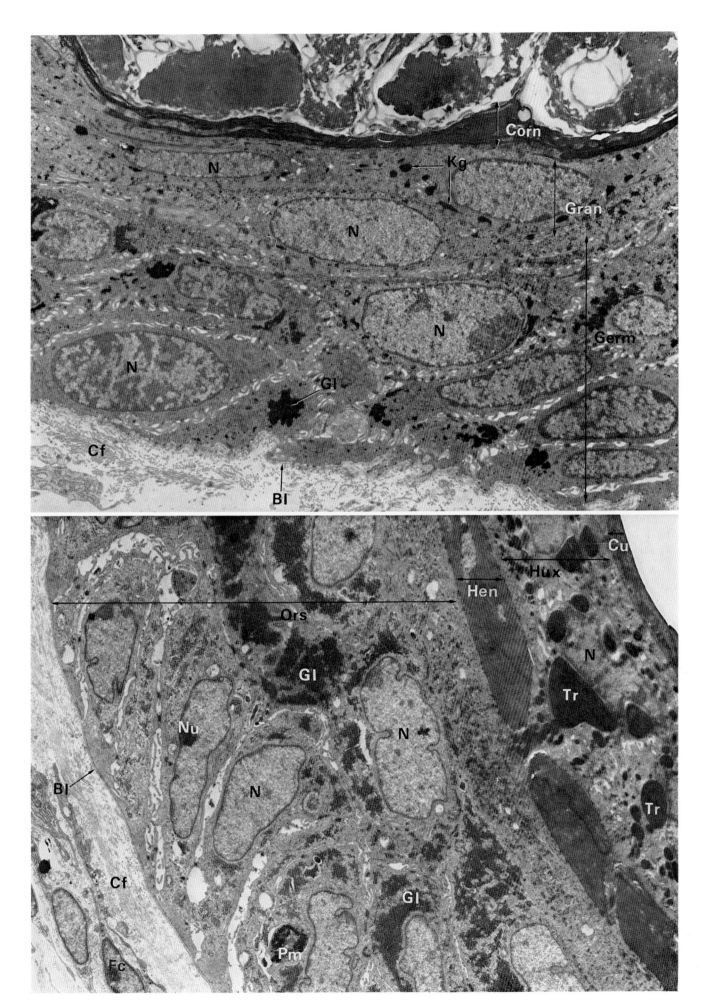

Sebaceous gland

The sebaceous gland is located superficially in the dermis, appended to the outer root sheath of the hair follicle. The oily product of this gland, sebum, consists of the degenerated cells of the gland filled with fat droplets.

Top : This micrograph shows a cluster of the epithelial cells of a sebaceous gland. The mature cells have a central nucleus (N) and numerous lipid droplets (Ld) in the cytoplasm. The droplets appear vacuolar because of the extraction of the contents in the course of fixation and dehydration, but a small amount of flocculent material remains. The cell border is provided with numerous short foldings partly interdigitated with those of the adjacent cells. Undifferentiated cells (Uc) situated in the peripheral portion are squamous in shape. They contain no lipid droplet and are similar in appearance to the cells of outer root sheath (Ors).

> Cf : Collagenous fiber.
> Fc : Fibrocyte.
> Hs : Hair shaft.

Bottom : Portions of sebaceous cells enclosed by the rectangle in the top micrograph. The sebaceous cell is, in its developing stage, usually provided with abundant profiles of smooth-surfaced endoplasmic reticulum which is intimately related to the formation of lipid. In the cells shown in this micrograph, such a structure is not clearly discernible. Scattered profiles of granular endoplasmic reticulum and numerous free ribosomes occur in the cytoplasm. Cytoplasmic foldings of the cell surface are clearly shown.

> d : Desmosome.
> Ld : Lipid droplet.
> m : Mitochondrion.
> N : Nucleus.
> Ors : Cell of the outer root sheath.

Top and Bottom : Material and method are the same as those of the pictures on page 255. Top : ×2,500. Bottom : ×12,000.

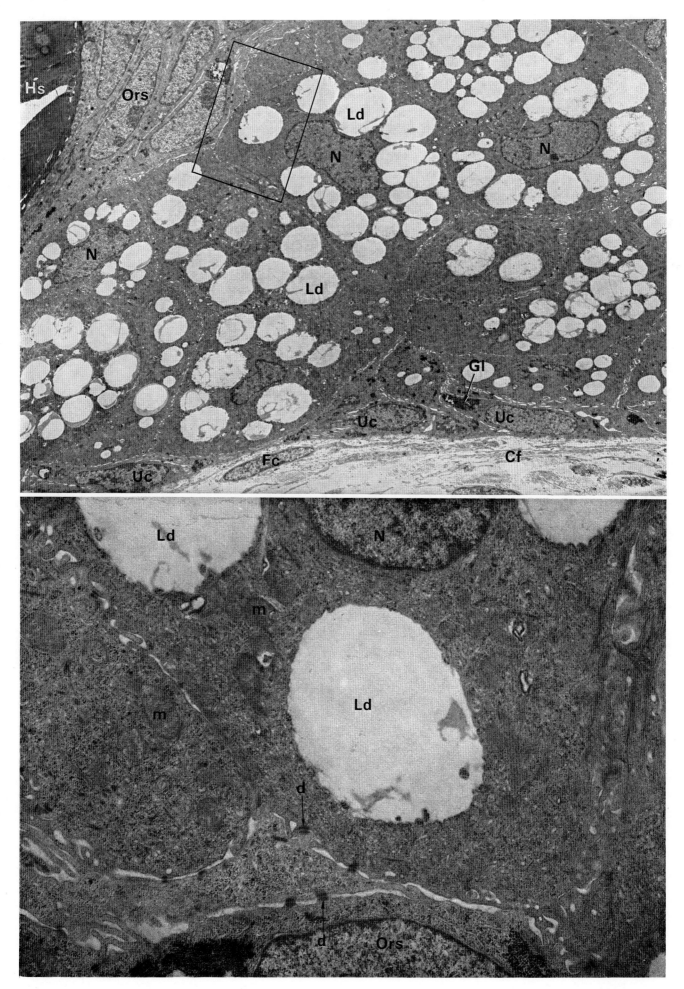

Secretory portion of the eccrine sweat gland

The sweat gland is an unbranched, coiled tubular gland whose secretory portion lies deep in the dermis or in the subcutaneous tissue.

This micrograph shows profiles of the secretory portion of the sweat gland. The secretory portion consists of single-layered glandular cells invested by myoepithelial cells (Mc). There are three types of glandular cells. The first type (T_1) is the cell characterized by the presence of numerous, dense granules (g) which are thought to contain a mucous substance. The second type cell (T_2) contains no granules. As it appears identical with the first type in other respects, it is thought to represent a different functional stage of the first type. The third type cell (T_3) is usually located in the basal side of the glandular epithelium and does not reach the glandular lumen. However, intercellular canaliculi (Ic) which empty into the glandular lumen are formed between adjacent cells of this type. The lateral cell surfaces exhibit complicated interdigitations. Glycogen particles (Gl) are rich in the cytoplasm. This type of cell is thought to take part in the production of water and salts of sweat.

The myoepithelial cells (Mc) are specialized smooth muscle cells which lie between the secretory epithelial cells and basal lamina (Bl). By their contraction, they contribute to the discharge of secretion from the sweat gland.

Collagenous fibers (Cf) surround the outside of the basal lamina. Bundles of non-myelinated nerve fibers (Nf) are seen in the space between profiles of secretory portions.

Glu: Glandular lumen.
Go: Golgi complex.
Ld: Lipid droplet.

Biopsy material obtained for diagnostic purpose from the upper arm of a 3-year-old female with urticaria pigmentosa. Method for specimen preparation is the same as that of the picture on page 243. ×7,000.

Hibbs, R. G.: The fine structure of human eccrine sweat glands. Amer. J. Anat., *103*: 201–217, 1958.

Ito, T. and S. Shibasaki: Electron microscopic study on human eccrine sweat glands. Arch. histol. jap., *27*: 81–115, 1966.

Kurosumi, K., T. Kitamura and K. Kano: Electron microscopy of the human eccrine sweat gland from an aged individual. Arch. histol. jap., *20*: 253–269, 1960.

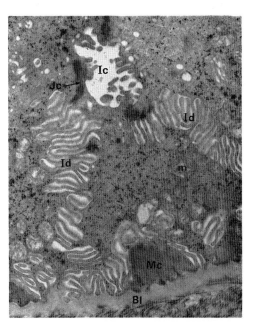

Intercellular canaliculus of the secretory portion of the sweat gland

Several microvilli are provided on the free surfaces bordering the canalicular lumen (Ic). The adjacent cells are attached by a junctional complex (Jc) near the lumen. Note the thick basal lamina (Bl) and extensive interdigitations (Id).

Material and method are the same as those of the picture on page 259. ×18,000.

258

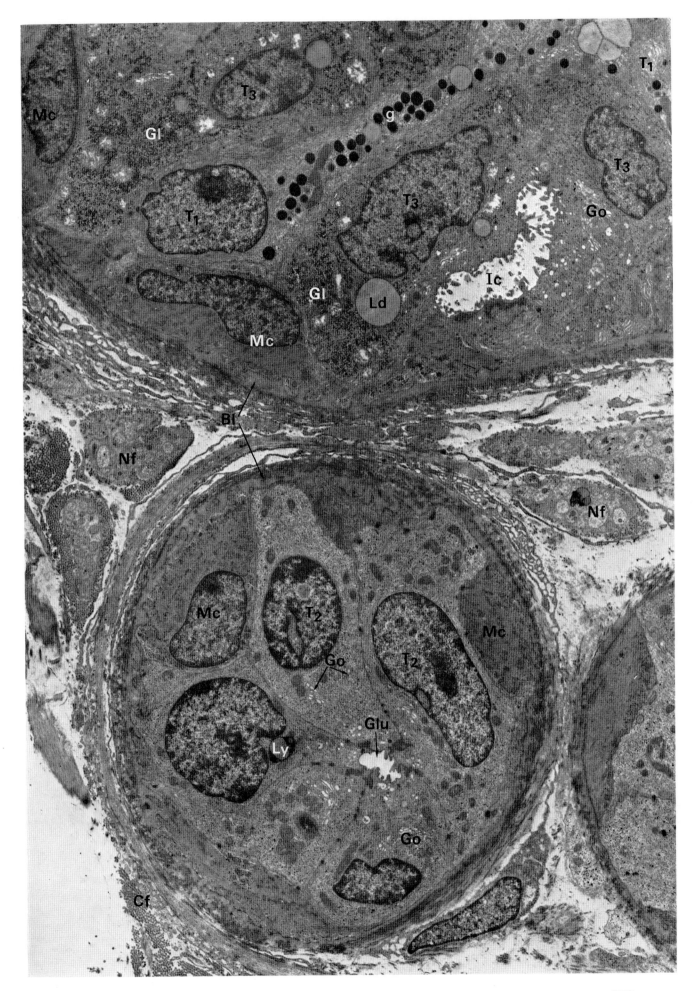

259

Sweat duct in the dermis

The secretory portion of the sweat gland empties into the excretory duct which continues through the epidermis to the free surface. In the dermis the duct is spiral in course and consists of two layers of cuboidal cells, but the intraepidermal portion is merely a cleft-like tunnel bordered by concentrically arranged keratinocytes. Myoepithelial cells do not occur in the duct.

This micrograph shows a section of a sweat duct in the dermis. The surface cells (Sc) border the duct lumen (Dlu). The cytoplasm subjacent to the free surface looks dense due to the condensation of tonofilaments. Numerous vacuoles are present beneath this area. The supranuclear cytoplasm exhibits relatively high density because of the presence of numerous tonofilaments. The lateral cell membranes form numerous interdigitations (Id). Desmosomes frequently occur here.

The basal cells (Bc) are located between the surface cells and the basal lamina (Bl). They contain many mitochondria and a large number of glycogen particles (Gl).

Cap : Capillary.
Fc : Fibrocyte.
Ly : Lysosome.

Surgically obtained abdominal skin of a 61-year-old male with esophageal cancer. Fixation with 2.0% glutaraldehyde followed by post-fixation with 1.0% osmium tetroxide solution. Uranyl acetate and lead tartarate staining. ×4,000.

REFERENCE:

SHIBASAKI, S. and T. ITO: Electron microscopic study on the duct of the human eccrine sweat gland with special remarks on the transitional portion epithelium. Arch. histol. jap., *28*: 285–312, 1967.

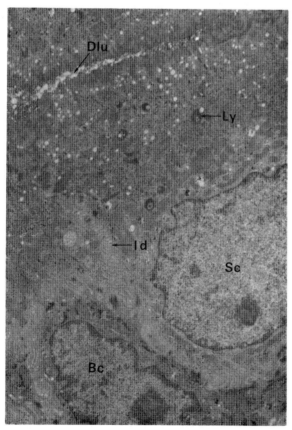

A portion of the sweat duct
Abbreviations are the same as for the picture on page 261.

Material and method are the same as those of the picture on page 261. ×10,000.

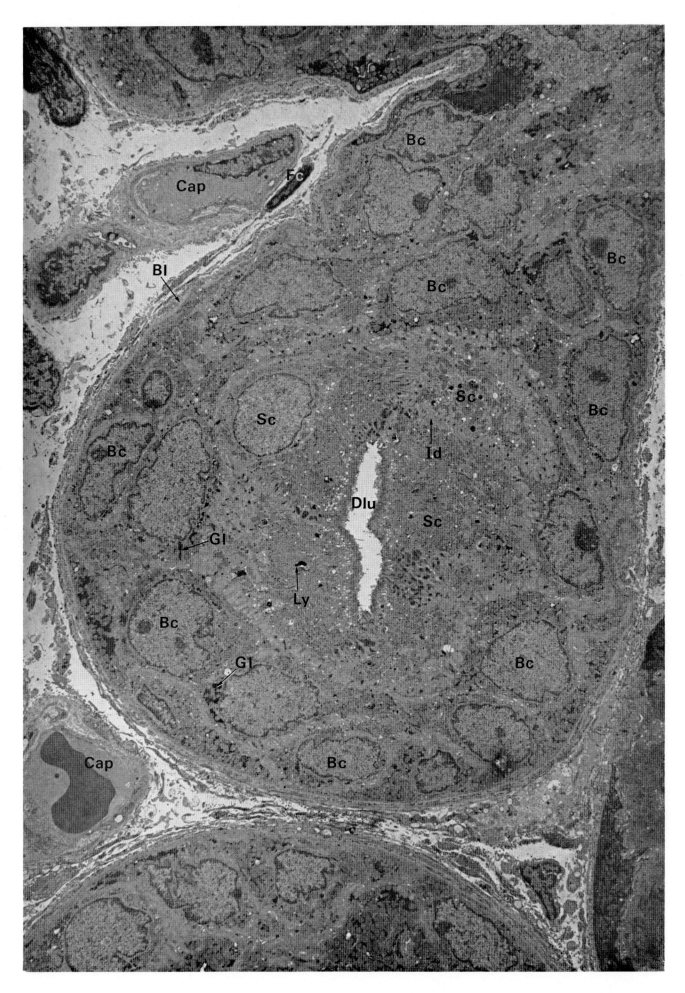

Secretory portion of the lactating mammary gland

The mammary gland is a modified sweat gland. Although it is present in both sexes, full differentiation and function are attained only in the woman after child-birth. Electron microscope studies revealed that the lipid in the milk is released by a type of apocrine secretion, whereas the proteinic components such as casein are released by reverse pinocytosis.

This electron micrograph shows the secretory portion of a lactating mammary gland. This portion consists of a single layer of glandular cells (Gc) and a discontinuous layer of myopithelial cells (Mc). The glandular cells are low columnar in shape and extend from the lumen (Lu) to the basal lamina (Bl). Several short microvilli (Mv) project from the luminal surfaces of the cells into the glandular lumen. The lateral surfaces are, as is common in epithelial cells, firmly attached to each other near the lumen by junctional complexes (Jc). The nucleus (N) of the glandular cell is situated toward the base of the cell and possesses a moderate amount of chromatin in its periphery. In the cytoplasm are scattered a large number of lipid droplets (Ld), distended cisterns of granular endoplasmic reticulum (Er), mitochondria (m) and numerous lysosomes (Ly). A Golgi complex (Go) occurs in the supranuclear region. Although membrane-bound secretory granules, considered to correspond to a proteinic component of the milk, are usually seen in the glandular cells, they are not distinct in this picture.

In the left center of this micrograph, there is an intercellular canalicule (Ic). It is formed by two adjacent glandular cells and sealed from the intercellular space by junctional complexes (Jc). The cell membrane bordering the canalicule bears many microvilli. As there seems to be no report on the occurrence of the intercellular canalicule in animal mammary glands, this may be a characteristic feature of the human material.

Between glandular cells and the basal lamina are myoepithelial cells (Mc). Most of their cytoplasm is occupied by fine filaments identical with those of the smooth muscle fibers. The myoepithelial cells contract to squeeze out the milk in response to nervous and hormonal stimuli.

Surgically-obtained lactating mammary gland of a 37-year-old female who was diagnosed as having a breast cancer about one year after her last child-birth. Veronal-buffered 1.0% osmium tetroxide fixation. Uranyl acetate and lead citrate staining. ×11,000. (Photograph courtesy of Drs. K. KUROSUMI and N. BABA)

REFERENCE:

WAUGH, D. and E. VAN DER HOEVEN: Fine structure of the human adult female breast. Lab. Invest., *11*: 220–228, 1962.

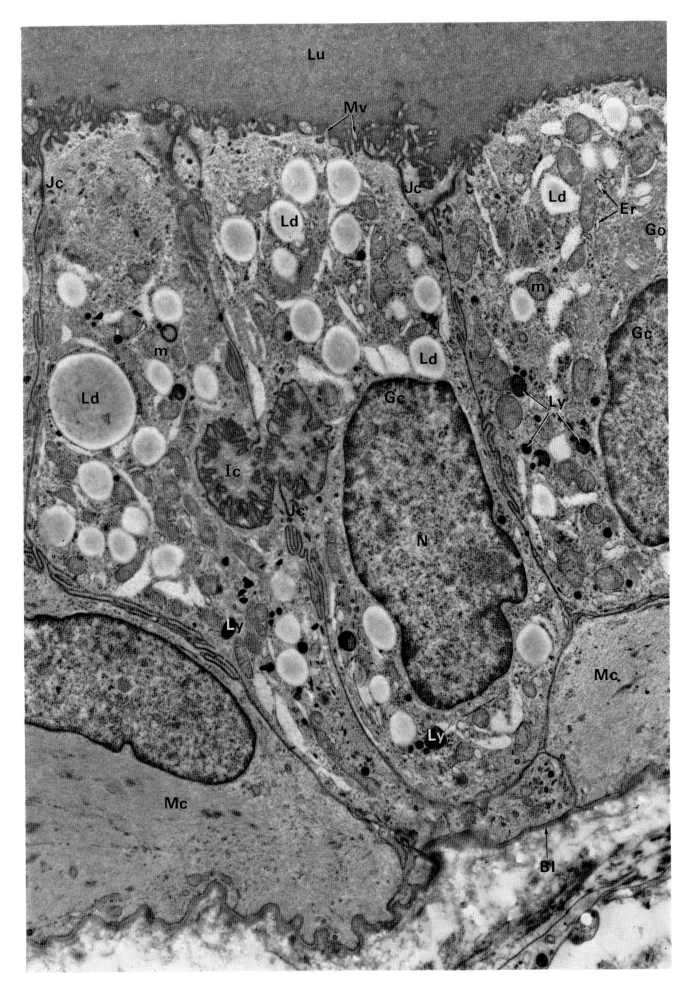

INDEX